Table of Contents

THE FOREARM AND HAND

THE SHOULDER GIRDLE AND ARM

THE LEG AND FOOT

THE HIP GIRDLE AND THIGH

THE NON-LIMB MUSCLES

Dedication

This work is dedicated to:

- James W. Albers, MD, PhD, from the University of Michigan, my mentor in the area of electromyography, who first inspired me to transform my daily teaching of anatomy into a published work;
- Karen Bantel, PhD, my wife, and David, Jeffrey, and Brian, my sons;
- My mother and father, who died 8 weeks apart in the fall of 1991.

My deep appreciation and respect go to Shayne Davidson, medical illustrator and my colleague in this work, whose professionalism and standards of excellence played a primary role in the successful completion of *Anatomic Localization*.

Foreword

As a fledgling electromyographer, I experienced my greatest anxiety with the needle electrode examination. Some of this anxiety reflected the anticipated discomfort the patient would experience during the examination, but most related to the anticipated discomfort I would experience learning sufficient peripheral anatomy to perform the examination. Like most physicians, I remember my experience as a first-year medical student memorizing the muscles and their insertions, actions, and innervations. I soon realized that the knowledge necessary to perform an EMG examination was very different from that needed to identify a muscle with a string around it in the anatomy laboratory and a label inquiring "What is this?" Detailed descriptions of muscle insertions, innervations, and actions did not help localize the brachialis muscle when I was uncertain of proper electrode insertion. I was fortunate to have mentors who were sensitive to these anxieties and experienced in teaching the art of needle examination.

When I began to teach clinical electromyography to others, I discovered the difficulty of this task. At the same time, I developed a greater understanding of peripheral anatomy as I tried to teach others how to perform a needle electrode examination. Much of that understanding occurred while "teaching" EMG to Dr. Geiringer. I discovered that he was a student of anatomy who understood three-dimensional relationships and who could use this knowledge in the EMG laboratory. His skills derived from hours of anatomical dissection, and many of our discussions based upon my "opinions" found resolution in the anatomy laboratory, resulting in modification of my opinions. His practical application of basic anatomy soon became the standard within our EMG laboratory, and his bedside lectures were formalized into a handout for the residents. This practical handbook of *Anatomic Localization for Needle Electromyography* is a graphic extension of the method successfully used by Dr. Geiringer to teach hundreds of students, residents, and associates over the past 10 years.

The material contained in this handbook addresses many of the anxieties I experienced initially as a resident, but even later as a more experienced electromyographer. Like others, I learned that patient discomfort corresponds inversely with the skill and confidence of the electromyographer. Choosing needle insertion sites that are less sensitive than others, advancing the electrode parallel to the muscle fibers using crisp, discrete movements, avoiding endplate regions, discouraging vigorous contractions with the electrode in place, and informing the patient throughout the study are all important steps in reducing physical and emotional discomfort. However, recognize that one of the clearest ways to increase patient anxiety and discomfort is to increase your own anxiety. Plunging the electrode into a patient's forearm and then anxiously searching for a specific muscle, discovering that the intended action results in electrical silence, produce the spiral of unexpected technical difficulty, eroded confidence, and patient intolerance. The increased physician and patient anxiety makes it difficult, if not impossible, to obtain the information required to complete the electrodiagnostic examination.

As with any procedure, proper technique is a prerequisite for interpretation of the derived information. The best clinician does make the best electromyographer, but only insofar as the examination is performed with sufficient skill to obtain the information required to confirm a diagnosis. Knowing where to put the EMG electrode seems like a trivial first step, but it is the most fundamental knowledge required to initiate the diagnostic process. Misinformation based upon improper electrode placement represents a common form of technical error easily corrected.

This is not a handbook on the differential diagnosis of neuromuscular diseases or a handbook on electrodiagnostic medicine. Instead, it is a practical description of the needle examination based upon identifiable landmarks and understanding of musculoskeletal anatomy, not on palpation of volitional contracted muscle. Dr. Geiringer correctly argues that the standard technique of asking the patient to contract the desired muscle is of little use in the uncooperative patient or the patient with limited or no movement. Under these circumstances, being able to identify a muscle using anatomic landmarks is essential for proper localization. His philosophy of visualizing the underlying anatomy and the path of the electrode is well demonstrated in this handbook of anatomic localization. Most electromyographers become comfortable with a limited number of muscles, modifying only the specific selection or the order of evaluation to solve particular problems. This illustrated guide permits even the experienced electromyographer to increase the repertoire of muscles for study. A current pocket handbook of medicine describes itself as containing all the information the residents need "at their fingertips." This is an appropriate description for this handbook of anatomic localization. All the information you need for your fingertips to perform an efficient, well-tolerated needle electrode examination exists within its covers.

JAMES W. ALBERS, MD, PhD
Professor of Neurology
Director, Neuromuscular Program and
 Electromyography Laboratory
University of Michigan Medical Center
Ann Arbor, Michigan

Introduction

The practice of electrodiagnostic medicine is inextricably linked to the science and art of human anatomy. Each practitioner draws from a substantial reservoir of knowledge during an EMG examination. Filling that reservoir, during years of residency training and later, can be a challenge to those of us not schooled as anatomists. This handbook is designed to facilitate the incorporation of anatomic principles into the practice of EMG. It is intended to be useful to students at all stages of learning, from residents in their first exposure to the electrodiagnostic laboratory, to the seasoned practitioner.

The approach to anatomic localization presented here arose from my teaching resident physicians in physical medicine and rehabilitation and neurology in the EMG laboratory at the University of Michigan in the early 1980s. My primary goal was to impart the basic principles of anatomy; the next step, i.e., where to place the needle in a real patient, followed naturally. Slides were made for lecture purposes; later, a lengthy handout was incorporated into the material given to each resident or fellow starting out in the laboratory. Dr. Jim Albers, the director of the lab at Michigan and my mentor in EMG, encouraged me early on to formalize this work as a publication unto itself. Nearly 10 years later, that has finally happened.

There is a subtle but important difference between the approach inherent in this handbook and those found elsewhere. This manual relies on, rather than substitutes for, knowledge of the basic principles of musculoskeletal anatomy, including the ability to visualize the muscles as they would appear under the skin and in cross-section. When the needle electrode is inserted into the patient, one should "see" its path as it passes through superficial structures, then approaches and enters the target muscle. Exactly where on the skin surface the needle enters is therefore of critical importance. Relying on fixed distances from bony landmarks quickly fails; a centimeter or the width of your finger will not serve you well if one patient is an infant or small adult and the next is a basketball player. Only a detailed knowledge of anatomy, including the three-dimensional relationships among muscles and bones which do not vary by patient, allows the electromyographer to consistently be confident of needle electrode placement in all patients.

While anatomy can be studied from textbooks, cadaver dissection at regular intervals is essential to bring this study "to life." This practice is strongly encouraged, especially with the needle electrode in hand, on a yearly basis if possible.

Other pitfalls of needle electromyography can be avoided by applying a working knowledge of anatomy. Some physicians early in training will start a needle examination by palpating the general area, asking the patient to contract the target muscle, palpating again, then inserting the electrode, and finally testing placement by asking for another voluntary contraction. It is important not to rely on this practice for the following reasons:

- A patient might not be able to activate a muscle voluntarily. This could result from nerve injury, hemiparesis, coma, upper motor neuron disorders, hysteria, or other factors.
- Some muscles might not be palpable in the obese patient.
- Patients tend to be most comfortable with the briefest test possible. Palpation, contraction, and repalpation take time, small increments of which extend the length of an examination.
- The patient's confidence in the examiner, crucial for a successful electrodiagnostic evaluation, might be compromised if as much time is spent searching for a muscle as examining it.
- Voluntary contraction to verify placement can be misleading, as contiguous muscles often have similar actions. The electrode might be mistakenly placed in the flexor carpi radialis muscle, for example, more distal than the intended pronator teres. Testing needle placement with forearm pronation will not reveal the error, as both muscles perform this function.
- Above all, one needs to be absolutely certain of the muscle being examined.

This manual is divided into five sections: forearm and hand, shoulder girdle and arm, leg and foot, hip girdle and thigh, and non-limb muscles. Within each section, representative muscles used in routine and specialized needle EMG examinations are included. No attempt has been made, however, to include every muscle potentially examined in electromyography. For example, upper and middle portions of the trapezius muscle are described, but not the approach to the lower trapezius muscle. Many deep-lying foot intrinsic muscles are omitted. Virtually any muscle, however, can be reliably isolated and examined if the corresponding anatomy is visualized.

The illustrations attempt to portray each muscle and its surrounding structures in the position recommended for examination, e.g., forearm in supination, side-lying, etc. In some cases, however, the orientation is influenced by the available space on the page, to display the pertinent anatomy optimally.

During the process of preparing this handbook, I have learned that no single illustration is able to convey all possible information about any muscle. For some (e.g., posterior tibialis), cross-sections or multiple views added to the existing drawing would be ideal. For others (e.g., supinator), superficial landmarks, such as the skin groove between two muscles, are not easily illustrated in the same drawing as the underlying muscle itself. My choice was to respect the limit of one illustration for each muscle, knowing that this occasionally results in compromise. The reader is once again encouraged to consider this work a starting point.

The listed root levels for each muscle were chosen after review of numerous anatomy and EMG references, combined with my own clinical experience. Any root level that is felt to supply primary innervation to a muscle is underlined. If two or more root levels are listed without underlining, each is felt to contribute nearly equally.

There is usually more than one method of reaching any muscle; I have found those detailed here to be the most reliable. Also, the recommended insertion points occasionally take into account such factors as the dorsal skin being thinner and less painful to pierce than the ventral skin. References to that and other hints are included throughout.

Once the correct insertion point is found, the monopolar or concentric needle electrode is inserted nearly parallel to the skin and along the muscle fiber orientation, which causes less pain than a perpendicular approach. Only rarely is that approach not possible (e.g., with iliopsoas or the paraspinal muscles). In the few muscles where the illustrated insertion point corresponds to the known motor endplate, this oblique angle of needle entry results in the endplate being "missed." Also, before asking for a voluntary contraction after studying insertional activity, you should pull the electrode fully back into the subcutaneous tissue. Enter only a lightly contracting muscle; a sudden, strong contraction with the electrode inserted can cause severe pain and can bend the needle.

As with other bodies of knowledge, if principles of anatomy are not continually used during EMG, they will be lost. On the other hand, if the principles outlined in this handbook can be incorporated into everyday practice, they will become second nature, and the resulting needle EMG examinations will be efficient and well tolerated.

STEVE R. GEIRINGER, MD
Associate Professor of Physical Medicine
   and Rehabilitation
Wayne State University
The Rehabilitation Institute of Michigan
Detroit, Michigan

How to Use This Book

The descriptions of anatomic localization contained in this book are meant to supplement, not substitute for, a thorough understanding of musculoskeletal anatomy. Included for each muscle are its *peripheral nerve supply* and *root level* of innervation. If a root level is felt to represent a primary source of innervation, it is underlined. If two or more root levels are listed without underlining, each is felt to contribute nearly equally. The illustrations depict the recommended *patient position* or limb position and, where appropriate, placement of the examiner's fingers. Whenever possible, the drawings are oriented on the page as the patient or limb would be viewed by the practitioner in the EMG laboratory. *Localization* includes a written description to help you visualize the pertinent bony or soft tissue landmarks and to guide you to a specific point on the skin for electrode insertion, marked on each illustration with an X. Because anatomic terms are used, rather than fixed distances or fingerbreadths, the instructions are applicable to patients of any size. Once the needle is through the skin, each description will aid in visualizing its path, whether through or past other muscles, against bones, or past neurovascular structures, until the targeted muscle is reached. *Activation* describes the maneuver used to elicit a voluntary contraction. *Cautions* are often added, usually noting nearby muscles which might be mistakenly entered. Finally, *notes* are added for most muscles, which pertain to clinical correlates, anatomic variations, or other points.

THE
FOREARM
AND
HAND

Abductor Digiti Quinti (hand)

PERIPHERAL NERVE   Ulnar

ROOT LEVELS   C8, T1

PATIENT POSITION   Arm at side, hand pronated.

LOCALIZATION   Directly at the medial border of the hand, at the midpoint between the distal wrist crease and the metacarpophalangeal crease. It is the first muscle encountered.

ACTIVATION   Abduction of digit 5.

NOTE   1. Although the muscle is located directly medial, approach it from the dorsal side of the ulnar border of the hand. There, the thinner skin is less painful to pierce than directly at the border of the hand.
2. When the needle electrode is inserted obliquely through the skin, as recommended, the motor point is avoided.

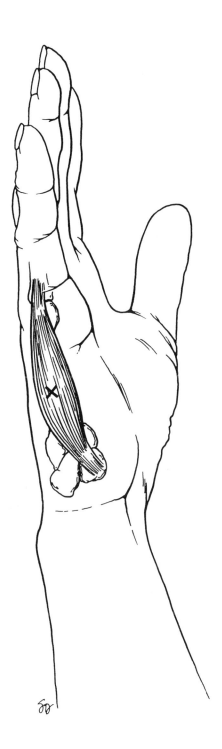

Abductor Pollicis Brevis

PERIPHERAL NERVE   Median

ROOT LEVELS   C8, T1

PATIENT POSITION   Arm at side, hand in supination.

LOCALIZATION   Parallel to first metacarpal shaft, in line with the mid-shaft of the extended first phalanx of the thumb, where it is the first muscle met by the electrode.

ACTIVATION   Abduction of thumb, i.e., movement of thumb out of the plane of the palm.

CAUTION   1. Do not stray too far from the radial edge of the thenar eminence. If the needle is too deep or too medial, it could be in flexor pollicis brevis, the deep head of which is ulnar innervated.
2. The ulnar-innervated adductor pollicis lies deep to the abductor pollicis brevis.

NOTE   1. The motor units in abductor pollicis brevis are generally easily recorded close to the surface. This muscle is painful to examine, so use no more than 1 cm of electrode length. The opponens pollicis is sometimes less painful to examine, as it can be approached through thinner, dorsal skin.
2. When the needle electrode is inserted obliquely through the skin, as recommended, the motor point is avoided.

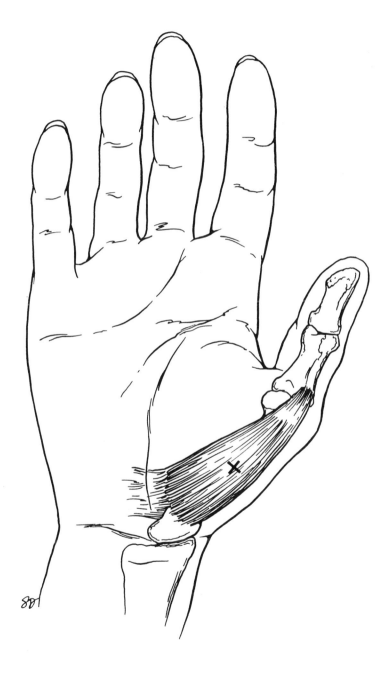

Abductor Pollicis Longus and Extensor Pollicis Brevis

PERIPHERAL NERVE   Posterior interosseous branch of radial nerve

ROOT LEVEL   C7, <u>C8</u>

PATIENT POSITION   Forearm fully pronated at the side.

LOCALIZATION   In the distal 25% of the dorsal forearm, overlying the radius.

ACTIVATION   Abduction and extension of the proximal phalanx of the thumb.

NOTE   1. Along with extensor pollicis longus, these are the thumb "outcropping" muscles, originating deep in the proximal forearm and becoming superficial distally.
2. The tendons of these two muscles form the ventral side of the anatomic snuff box at the radial side of the wrist.
3. The muscle bellies can be difficult to separate reliably. The abductor pollicis longus becomes superficial just proximal to the extensor pollicis brevis.

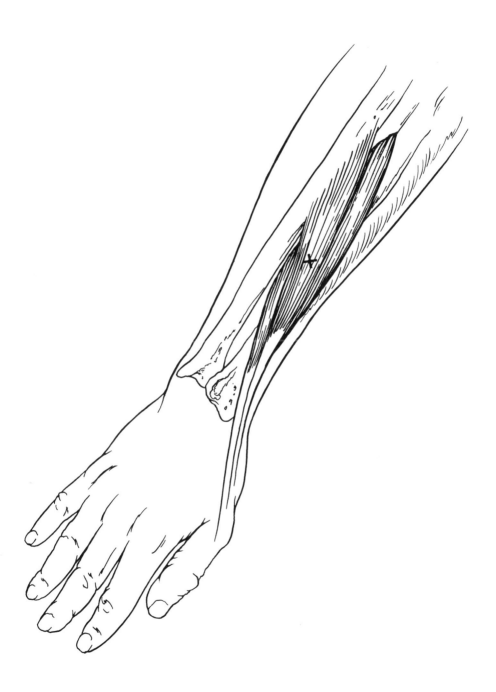

Adductor Pollicis

PERIPHERAL NERVE   Ulnar, deep palmar branch

ROOT LEVEL   C8, T1

PATIENT POSITION   Arm at side, hand resting on ulnar border, i.e., midway between pronation and supination.

LOCALIZATION   Immediately proximal to the first metacarpophalangeal joint, the electrode is inserted in the groove between the metacarpal bone and first dorsal interosseous muscle and toward the depth of the web space. At this fairly distal location, the bulk of the first dorsal is avoided.

ACTIVATION   Thumb adduction within the plane of the palm.

CAUTION   If the ulnar-supplied muscles in the web space are atrophic, the electrode could enter the median-innervated thenar muscles.

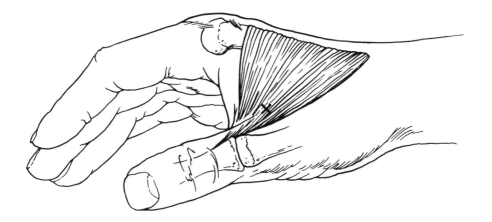

Anconeus

PERIPHERAL NERVE	Radial
ROOT LEVELS	<u>C7</u>, C8
PATIENT POSITION	Forearm in pronation, across abdomen.
LOCALIZATION	The electrode is inserted midway between the olecranon process and the lateral epicondyle. No other muscle is found at this location.
ACTIVATION	Elbow extension.
CAUTION	At a location more distal than recommended, the extensor carpi ulnaris lies adjacent (lateral) to anconeus. This muscle is also supplied by the radial nerve, although by the posterior interosseous branch.
NOTE	Anconeus is essentially a distal extension of the triceps and is the last muscle innervated by the radial nerve before the spiral groove of the humerus. It is therefore helpful in localizing spiral groove lesions.

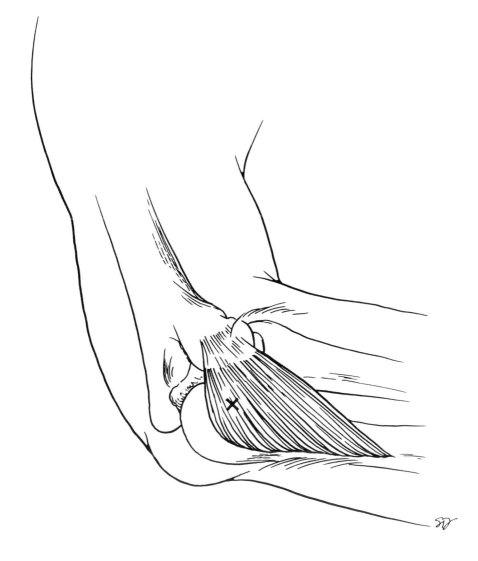

Brachioradialis

PERIPHERAL NERVE   Radial

ROOT LEVELS   C5, <u>C6</u>

PATIENT POSITION   Forearm fully supinated.

LOCALIZATION   Place index finger in the antecubital fossa, pointing proximal. Brachioradialis is the first muscle lateral to your finger.

ACTIVATION   Elbow flexion, with the forearm in mid pronation-supination.

CAUTION   If the needle electrode is placed too laterally, it could be in the radial wrist extensors.

NOTE   Brachioradialis is the first muscle innervated by the radial nerve after its course through the spiral groove; therefore, it can be helpful for localizing radial neuropathies.

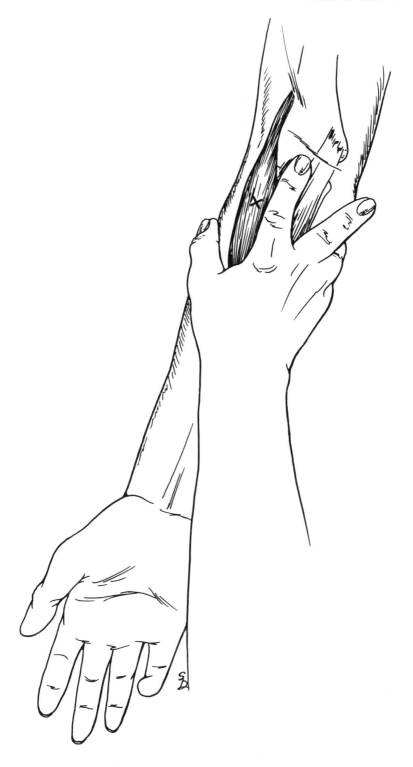

Extensors Carpi Radialis Brevis and Longus

PERIPHERAL NERVE   Radial

ROOT LEVELS   <u>C6</u>, C7

PATIENT POSITION   Forearm fully pronated, elbow flexed to 30°.

LOCALIZATION   Visualize the line connecting the lateral epicondyle and the radial styloid process. In the proximal half of the forearm, this line separates the extensor digitorum communis from the wrist extensors, with a groove between them. The extensors are therefore approached just lateral to this line (i.e., to the thumb side) and are superficial.

ACTIVATION   Wrist extension.

CAUTION   If the electrode is too lateral, it will be in the brachioradialis. If it is too medial, it will be in the extensor digitorum communis.

NOTE   The extensors carpi radialis brevis and longus are difficult to distinguish during the EMG examination. The long extensor is purely tendinous in the distal half of the forearm, whereas the muscle fibers of the short extensor persist farther distally. Additionally, extensor carpi radialis longus lies medial and ventral to the brevis.

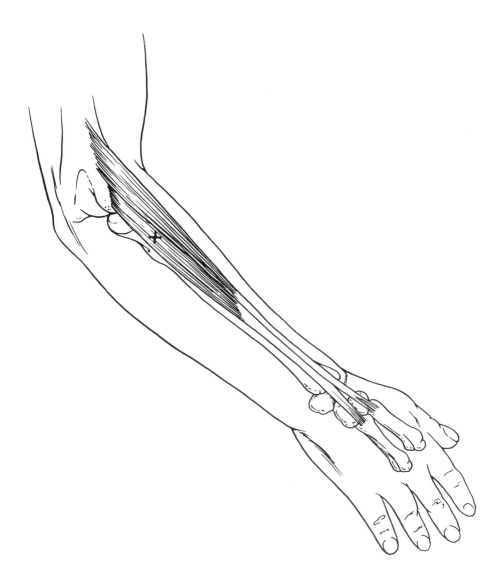

Extensor Carpi Ulnaris

PERIPHERAL NERVE   Posterior interosseous branch of radial nerve

ROOT LEVELS   C7, C8

PATIENT POSITION   Forearm fully pronated, or forearm lying across abdomen.

LOCALIZATION   In the proximal half of the forearm, just dorsal to the ulnar shaft, and superficial.

ACTIVATION   Wrist extension combined with ulnar deviation.

CAUTION   The electrode inserted too laterally (i.e., toward the thumb side) will be in extensor digitorum communis or extensor digiti minimi. If it is too deep, it will most likely be in one of the thumb outcropping muscles.

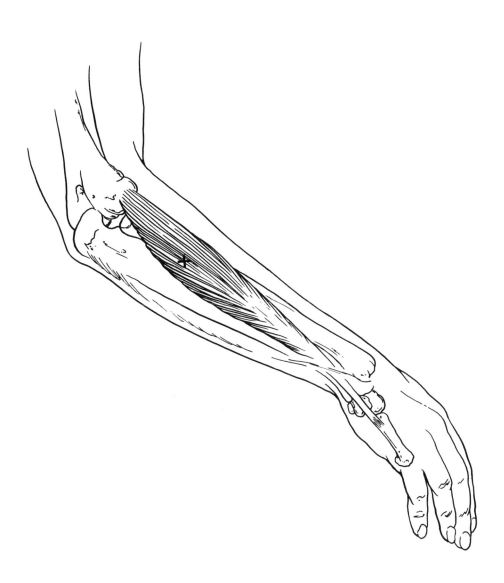

Extensor Digitorum Communis

PERIPHERAL NERVE	Posterior interosseous branch of radial nerve
ROOT LEVELS	C7, C8
PATIENT POSITION	Forearm fully pronated.
LOCALIZATION	Brachioradialis and the radial wrist extensors comprise a "movable mass" of muscles. Just medial to this group is a groove separating it from the extensor digitorum communis, which itself is relatively immovable. The division occurs in the proximal half of the forearm, along the line connecting the lateral epicondyle and radial styloid. The electrode is therefore inserted just medial to and parallel to that groove, in the proximal forearm, where the extensor digitorum communis is superficial.
ACTIVATION	Extension of digits 2 through 5.
CAUTION	If the needle is too lateral (i.e., toward the thumb side), it will be in the wrist extensors. If it is too medial, it can be in the extensor carpi ulnaris. Insertion too distal places it in the thumb extensors or the tendons of extensor digitorum communis.
NOTE	Extensor digitorum communis is the first muscle innervated by the posterior interosseous nerve after the nerve emerges from the supinator.

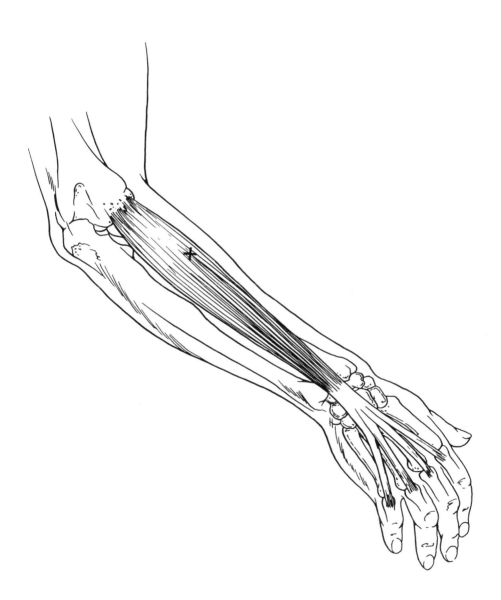

Extensor Indicis

PERIPHERAL NERVE   Posterior interosseous branch of radial nerve

ROOT LEVELS   C7, <u>C8</u>

PATIENT POSITION   Forearm fully pronated.

LOCALIZATION   In the distal 20% of the forearm, midway between the radius and ulna. At this distal location, extensor indicis is the only dorsal muscle that is not primarily tendinous.

ACTIVATION   Extension of the index finger.

CAUTION   The electrode inserted too proximally might enter extensor pollicis longus, which is muscular at this location and lies immediately adjacent (lateral) to extensor indicis.

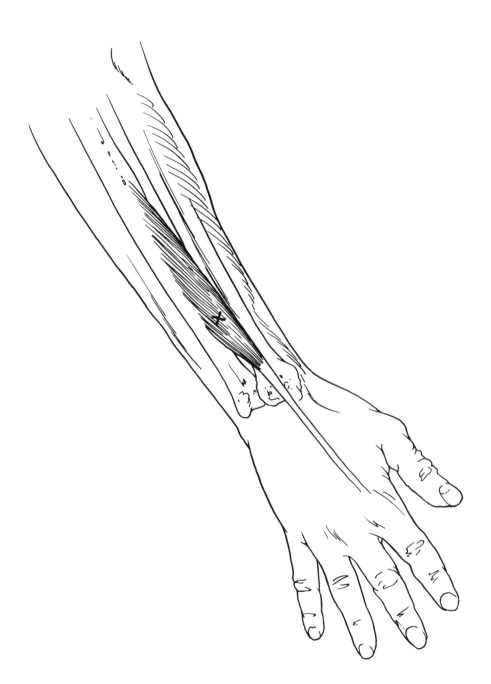

Extensor Pollicis Longus

PERIPHERAL NERVE   Posterior interosseous branch of radial nerve

ROOT LEVELS   C7, <u>C8</u>

PATIENT POSITION   Forearm fully pronated.

LOCALIZATION   Insert the electrode at the junction of the middle and lower thirds of the dorsal forearm, midway between the ulna and radius. At this point, extensor pollicis longus lies immediately beneath the distal muscle bellies of extensor digitorum communis.

ACTIVATION   Extension of distal phalanx of thumb.

CAUTION   If the needle electrode is placed too medially (toward the ulna), it will be in extensor indicis. If it is too lateral, it will in abductor pollicis longus.

NOTE   This muscle is difficult to isolate without verification by voluntary patient contraction. It lies deep and is bordered on three sides by other dorsal muscles.

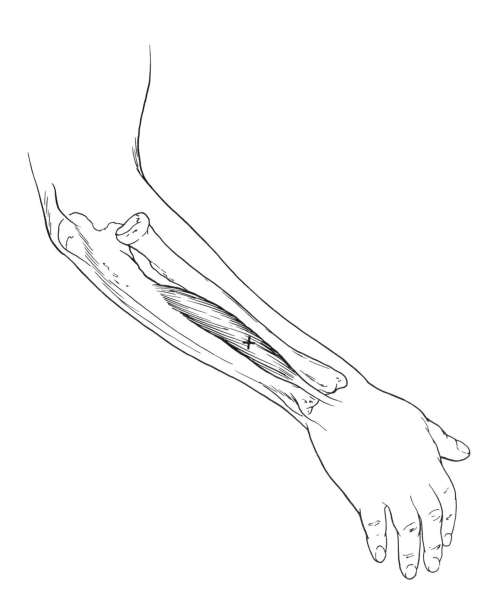

First Dorsal Interosseous (hand)

PERIPHERAL NERVE	Ulnar, deep palmar branch
ROOT LEVELS	C8, T1
PATIENT POSITION	Arm at side, forearm in neutral (i.e., midway between pronation and supination), resting on the ulnar border of the hand.
LOCALIZATION	The electrode is inserted parallel to the second metacarpal shaft, superficially, directly into the middle of the dorsal web space.
ACTIVATION	Abduction of digit 2 within the plane of the palm.
CAUTION	If the first dorsal interosseous is atrophic, the needle could enter adductor pollicis (also ulnar-innervated) or, less likely, the thenar group (mostly median-supplied).

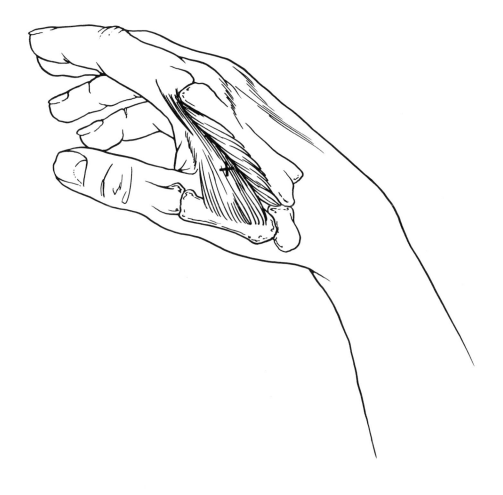

Flexor Carpi Radialis

PERIPHERAL NERVE   Median

ROOT LEVELS   C6, <u>C7</u>

PATIENT POSITION   Forearm fully supinated.

LOCALIZATION   Place index finger in the antecubital fossa, pointing proximal. Flexor carpi radialis is the first muscle medial to your finger at the level of the apex of the antecubital fossa (where brachioradialis and this muscle converge) and is superficial at that point.

ACTIVATION   Wrist flexion.

CAUTION   If the electrode is too proximal, it will be in pronator teres. If it is inserted too deeply or too medially, it will be in flexor digitorum superficialis.

NOTE   After diagnosing a median neuropathy at the wrist, it is wise to exclude a median nerve entrapment in the forearm (double crush). Flexor carpi radialis is more suited for this purpose than pronator teres, as pronator syndrome typically involves the former and spares the latter.

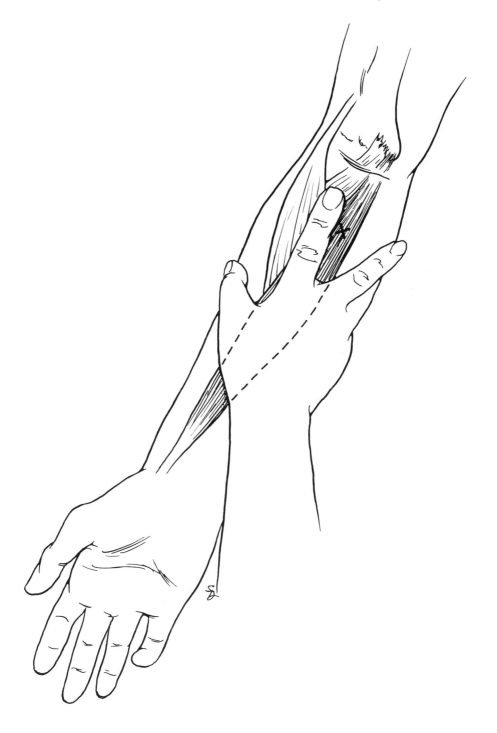

Flexor Carpi Ulnaris

PERIPHERAL NERVE   Ulnar

ROOT LEVELS   C8, T1

PATIENT POSITION   Forearm fully supinated.

LOCALIZATION   Middle third of the forearm, superficial and directly medial.

ACTIVATION   Wrist flexion with ulnar deviation.

CAUTION   The needle electrode must be inserted directly at the medial border of the forearm. If too anterior, the most common mistake, it will be in flexor digitorum superficialis, a muscle innervated by the median nerve. In the distal forearm, the muscle becomes thinner and aponeurotic. It is important that the electrode not stray into the underlying flexor digitorum profundus (*see* note 1 below).

NOTE   1. The nerve branch to flexor carpi ulnaris (FCU) occasionally arises above the point of entrapment in ulnar neuropathies "at the elbow." Flexor digitorum profundus is always innervated below the entrapment in these situations. A normal needle EMG study of FCU therefore does not eliminate an ulnar neuropathy in the elbow region; ideally, both muscles are examined when this clinical question arises.
2. The FCU is often described as having C7 innervation. This occurs in a minority of people, usually because the ulnar nerve has received a contribution from the lateral cord. Otherwise, all ulnar-innervated muscles are C8/T1, from the lower trunk and medial cord.

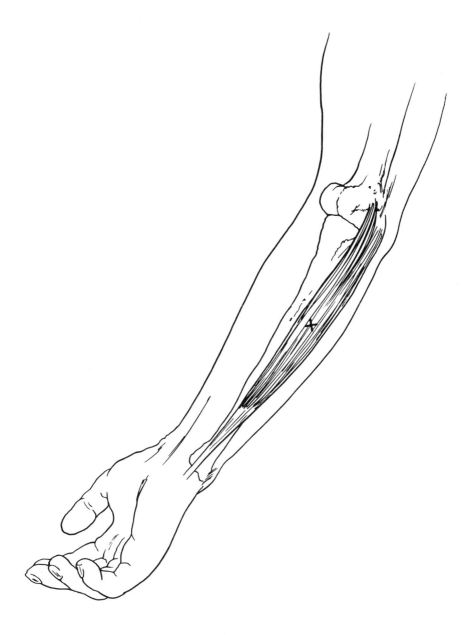

Flexor Digitorum Profundus, Ulnar (medial) Heads

PERIPHERAL NERVE   Ulnar

ROOT LEVELS   C8, T1

PATIENT POSITION   Forearm pronated and placed across the abdomen.

LOCALIZATION   In the middle one-third of the forearm, immediately ventral to the ulnar shaft. Here, the muscle lies just below the thin aponeurosis of flexor carpi ulnaris.

ACTIVATION   Flexion of the distal phalanges of digits 4 and 5.

NOTE

1. In the proximal forearm, the flexor territory is the medial one-half, not the ventral one-half; the extensor territory is the lateral half, not the dorsal. The ulnar shaft divides these territories posteriorly. The flexor digitorum profundus (FDP) is not easily reached with the forearm supinated, as the ulnar shaft will be directly against the table.

2. The branch of the ulnar nerve to FDP arises more distally than that to flexor carpi ulnaris, which occasionally arises above the level of ulnar entrapment "at the elbow." With ulnar neuropathies, it is therefore important to study FDP in addition to flexor carpi ulnaris.

3. The lateral heads of FDP, to digits 2 and 3, are supplied by the anterior interosseous branch of the median nerve. They lie in the deepest portion of the forearm and should be avoided on needle study if possible. If necessary, this portion of the muscle can be reached by inserting the electrode at mid-forearm, immediately lateral to flexor carpi radialis, directing it deep and medial. Localization needs to be verified with voluntary flexion of the corresponding distal phalanges. The radial artery might lie in the path of the advancing electrode.

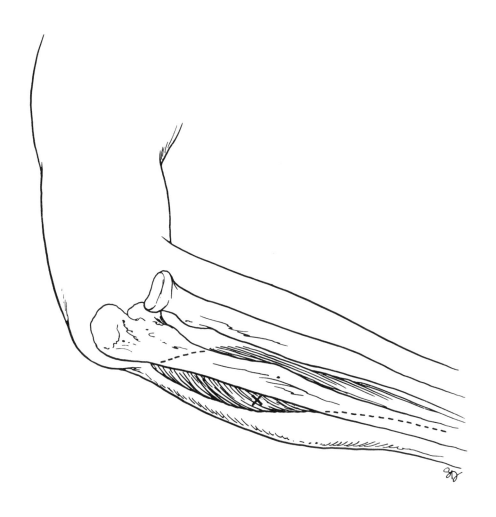

Flexor Digitorum Superficialis

PERIPHERAL NERVE Median

ROOT LEVELS C7, C8, T1

PATIENT POSITION Arm at side, forearm fully supinated.

LOCALIZATION At mid-forearm, halfway from the ventral midline to the medial border of the forearm. At this location, it is the first muscle reached.

ACTIVATION Finger or wrist flexion.

CAUTION 1. The electrode placed too medially will be in flexor carpi ulnaris.
2. The needle inserted too deeply will be in flexor digitorum profundus, the medial heads of which are supplied by the ulnar nerve.
3. The needle inserted too close to the ventral midline will be in flexor carpi radialis.

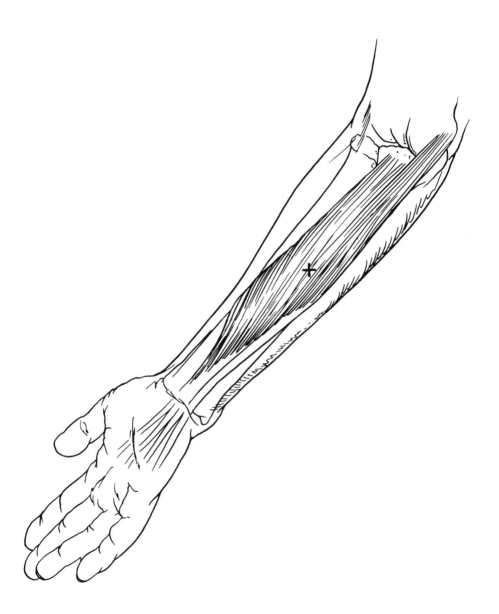

Flexor Pollicis Longus

PERIPHERAL NERVE Anterior interosseous branch of median nerve

ROOT LEVELS C7, <u>C8</u>

PATIENT POSITION Forearm in full supination.

LOCALIZATION In the middle of the ventral forearm, the electrode is inserted just distal to the convergence of the muscle bellies of flexor carpi radialis and brachioradialis, virtually at the midline—i.e., needle placement is just distal to the apex of the antecubital fossa. Direct the needle perpendicular to the skin and deep until bone is reached (the flat anterior surface of the radius). The last muscle traversed is flexor pollicis longus, so pull the needle out a few millimeters after reaching bone.

ACTIVATION Flexion of distal phalanx of thumb.

CAUTION 1. If the electrode is too medial, it will lie in the lateral heads of flexor digitorum profundus.
2. The radial artery is in the path of the advancing electrode.

NOTE 1. In anterior interosseous syndrome, flexor pollicis longus and pronator quadratus are somewhat more easily examined than the lateral heads of flexor digitorum profundus, although none of these muscles lies superficially at any point.
2. The outlines in the illustration indicate the superficial muscles used as landmarks for needle electrode insertion, flexor carpi radialis and brachioradialis.

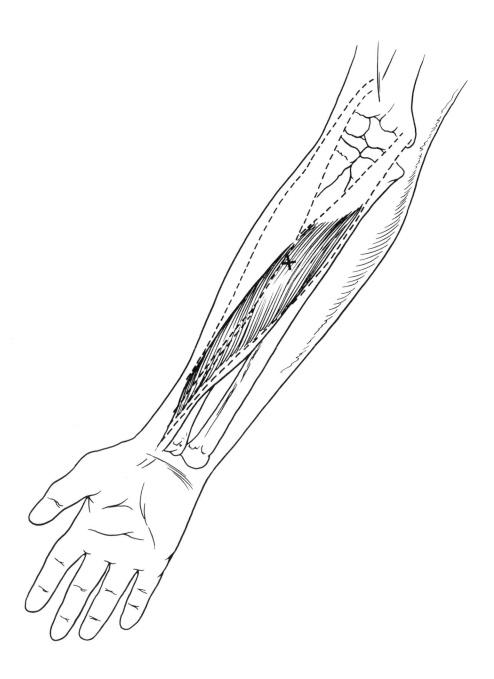

Opponens Pollicis

PERIPHERAL NERVE   Median

ROOT LEVELS   C8, T1

PATIENT POSITION   Hand in supination.

LOCALIZATION   At the midpoint of the first metacarpal shaft, in the groove between the metacarpal bone and abductor pollicis brevis. The muscle is studied where it attaches to the medial side of the bone. If abductor pollicis brevis is moved aside, no other muscle overlies the opponens at this point.

ACTIVATION   Opposition of thumb across the palm.

CAUTION   Once the muscle is reached, the needle should remain fairly superficial. If the electrode is inserted too deeply, it may be in the ulnar-innervated adductor pollicis.

NOTE   Opponens pollicis can be reached on needle examination through the thin skin of the dorsolateral thumb. This muscle tends to be less painful to examine, therefore, than the abductor pollicis brevis, which must be approached through the thick palmar skin.

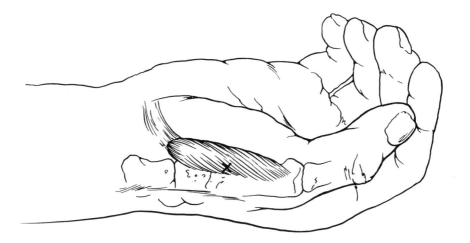

Pronator Quadratus

PERIPHERAL NERVE   Anterior interosseous branch of median nerve

ROOT LEVELS   C7, C8, T1

PATIENT POSITION   Arm at side, forearm fully supinated, wrist flexed.

LOCALIZATION   The muscle width is the same as its length, covering the distal 20% or so of the forearm, anterior to the interosseous membrane. Insert the electrode just anterior to the distal ulnar shaft, perpendicular to it, and direct the electrode horizontally to meet the thick medial border of the muscle.

ACTIVATION   Forearm pronation.

CAUTION   Without the wrist flexed, the ulnar nerve and artery can be in the path of the advancing electrode.

NOTE   1. This approach takes advantage of the fact that the anatomic origin of pronator quadratus (i.e., the medial side) is much thicker than its insertion into the radius.
2. It is less desirable to approach pronator quadratus directly from the ventral or dorsal forearm. On the ventral side, the median nerve lies directly in the path of the needle; on the dorsal side, extensor muscle tendons and the interosseous membrane must be traversed.

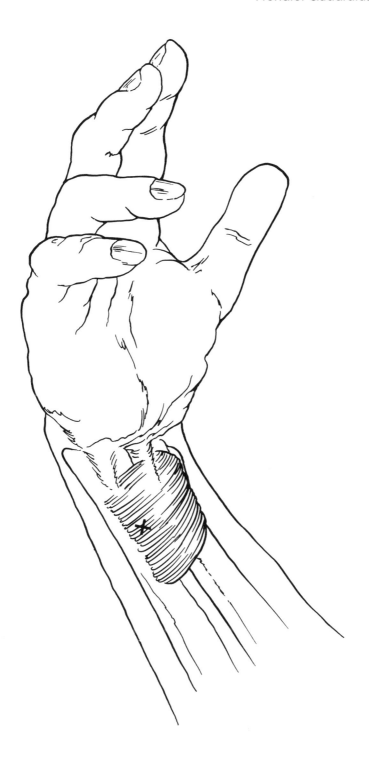

Pronator Teres

PERIPHERAL NERVE   Median

ROOT LEVELS   C6, C7

PATIENT POSITION   Forearm fully supinated.

LOCALIZATION   With the index finger in the antecubital fossa pointing proximal, pronator teres is the first muscle medial to your finger, immediately distal to the antecubital vein.

ACTIVATION   Elbow flexion or, if necessary, forearm pronation (*see* note 2 below).

CAUTION   A common mistake is for the electrode to be inserted too distal, in which case it will be in flexor carpi radialis. If the needle is inserted too medial, it will be in either flexor carpi ulnaris or flexor digitorum superficialis.

NOTE   1. Pronator teres is often used to rule out a proximal median neuropathy, e.g., pronator syndrome, when there is median compression at the wrist. Often, though, a muscle naming a syndrome is spared in that syndrome; e.g., the branch to pronator teres usually arises from the median nerve before the muscle entraps the nerve in pronator syndrome. Use flexor carpi radialis as a screen in this situation.
2. Pronator teres carries a strong secondary action of elbow flexion. This tends to be a less painful maneuver for voluntary activation than the primary function, forearm pronation.

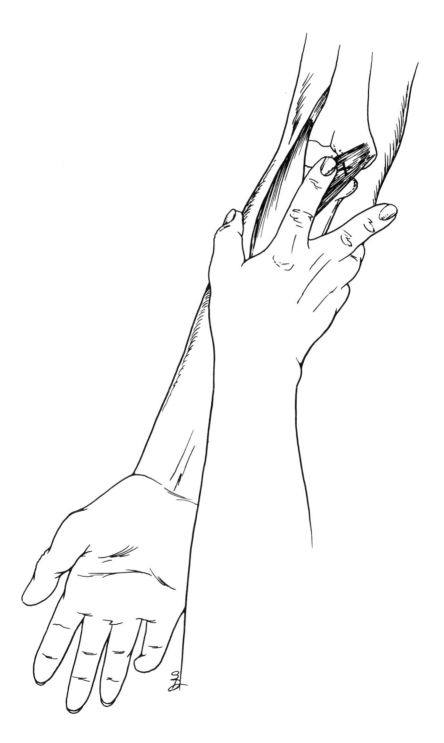

Supinator

PERIPHERAL NERVE	Radial
ROOT LEVELS	C5, <u>C6</u>
PATIENT POSITION	Forearm in pronation.
LOCALIZATION	In the proximal 20% of the dorsal forearm, insert the electrode in the groove between the radial wrist extensors (movable) and extensor digitorum communis (immovable). The electrode is directed deep, where supinator is found lying against the radius.
ACTIVATION	Forearm supination.
CAUTION	An alternative approach is from the medial border of brachioradialis, in the antecubital fossa. The radial artery and nerve might be encountered there, and the portion of supinator reached is thin.
NOTE	1. As in other nerve-entrapment syndromes named for a muscle, the supinator is often not affected in "supinator syndrome." Muscles supplied by the posterior interosseous nerve (e.g., extensor carpi ulnaris, extensor digitorum communis) can be examined to confirm this condition.
	2. The illustration depicts only the deep-lying supinator, not the superficial muscles used as landmarks for needle insertion.

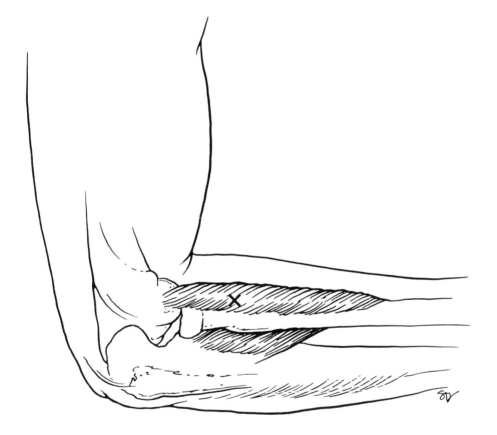

THE SHOULDER GIRDLE AND ARM

Biceps Brachii

PERIPHERAL NERVE   Musculocutaneous

ROOT LEVELS   C5, C6

PATIENT POSITION   Arm at side, elbow flexed 30°.

LOCALIZATION   Middle one-third of the arm, directly into and paralleling the muscle belly, approaching biceps from its lateral side.

ACTIVATION   Elbow flexion, with the forearm in supination.

NOTE   Motor unit recruitment is often difficult, as biceps is a two-joint muscle whose primary action is also carried by an underlying one-joint muscle, brachialis. Consider using brachialis if you have trouble recruiting motor units in biceps. Additionally, brachialis tends to be less painful for needle study than biceps.

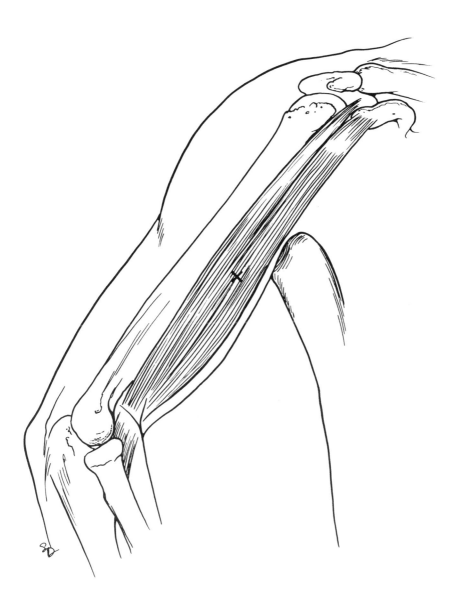

Brachialis

PERIPHERAL NERVE   Musculocutaneous

ROOT LEVELS   C5, C6

PATIENT POSITION   Arm at side, elbow flexed 30°.

LOCALIZATION   In the distal one-third of the arm, push the biceps medially and insert the electrode in the groove between biceps and triceps. Direct it down and medially, toward the anterior aspect of the humeral shaft.

ACTIVATION   Elbow flexion; the degree of forearm pronation-supination is irrelevant.

CAUTION   1. The biceps can be entered if it is not pushed far enough medially.
2. If the electrode is too posterior, it could be in triceps or the originating fibers of brachioradialis.
3. The cephalic vein could be pierced but usually lies anterior to the advancing electrode.
4. Brachialis usually receives a contribution from the radial nerve and occasionally from the median.

NOTE   Brachialis is easier to activate than biceps, because it is a one-joint muscle. Also, it tends to be less painful to test than biceps, as it can be approached through dorsal skin. Given their common nerve root and peripheral nerve supply, consider examining brachialis instead of biceps when either would do.

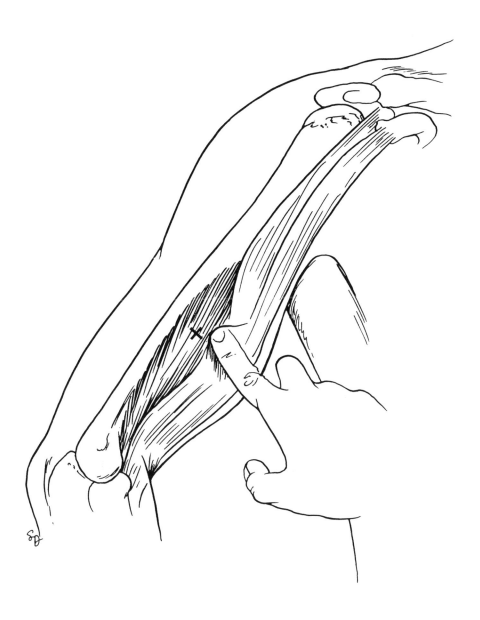

Deltoid, Anterior

PERIPHERAL NERVE Axillary

ROOT LEVELS C5, C6

PATIENT POSITION Side-lying or supine.

LOCALIZATION Midpoint of the line connecting the lateral one-third of the clavicle and the deltoid insertion.

ACTIVATION Arm abduction or shoulder flexion.

CAUTION The electrode inserted too anteriorly will be in pectoralis major, separated from deltoid by the cephalic vein.

NOTE Selective study of each portion of deltoid might be helpful (along with teres minor) when characterizing an axillary mononeuropathy.

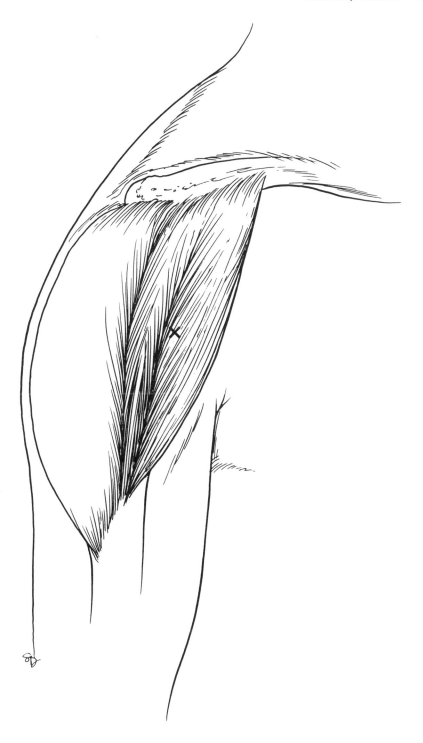

Deltoid, Middle

PERIPHERAL NERVE   Axillary

ROOT LEVELS   C5, C6

PATIENT POSITION   Supine, arm at side.

LOCALIZATION   One-third of the distance down the line between the acromion process and the deltoid insertion. Deltoid is the only muscle encountered in this location.

ACTIVATION   Arm abduction.

NOTE   The anterior or posterior fibers can be studied separately if needed, e.g., with an axillary mononeuropathy.

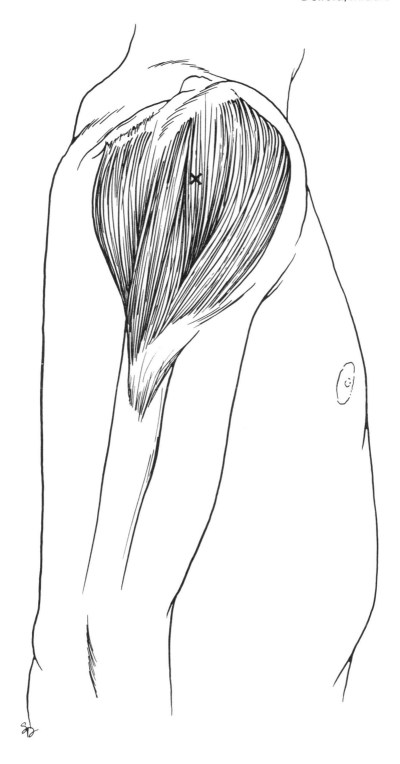

Deltoid, Posterior

PERIPHERAL NERVE   Axillary

ROOT LEVELS   C5, C6

PATIENT POSITION   Side-lying.

LOCALIZATION   Midpoint of the line connecting the distal scapular spine and the deltoid insertion.

ACTIVATION   Arm abduction or shoulder extension.

CAUTION   The electrode inserted too posteriorly could be in teres major or minor or the long head of triceps.

NOTE   Each head of deltoid might be studied separately when characterizing an axillary mononeuropathy.

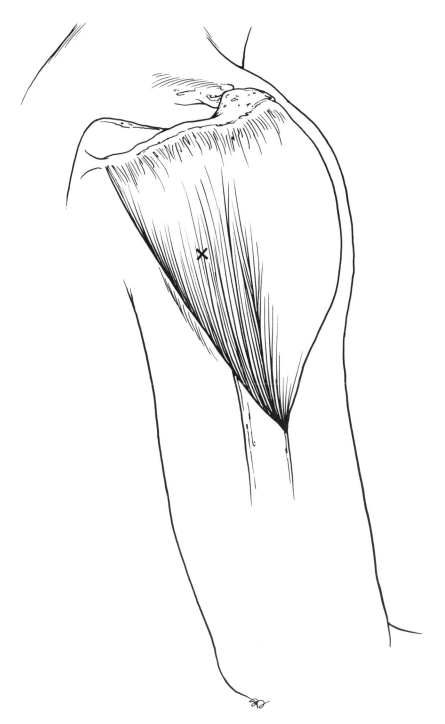

Infraspinatus

PERIPHERAL NERVE   Suprascapular

ROOT LEVELS   C5, C6

PATIENT POSITION   Side-lying on contralateral side, arm draped across front of body. Alternatively, lying prone.

LOCALIZATION   Halfway between the scapular spine and the inferior tip of the scapula, midway between the lateral and medial borders of the scapula—i.e., directly in the center of the infraspinous fossa. The electrode should first gently touch the posterior surface of the scapula, then be pulled back slightly to examine the infraspinatus.

ACTIVATION   External rotation of the arm. Activation is usually possible simply by the patient lifting the arm off the table.

CAUTION   Rarely, the lateral-most fibers of infraspinatus are innervated by the axillary nerve after it supplies teres minor. Avoid studying the lateral fibers of infraspinatus for this reason.

NOTE   Suprascapular nerve lesions usually occur either at the scapular notch under the transverse scapular ligament or at the scapular neck after supplying supraspinatus. Examining infraspinatus will serve as a screen for entrapment at either of these locations in patients with ill-defined shoulder pain. If a suprascapular palsy is clinically suspected, both spinati should be studied.

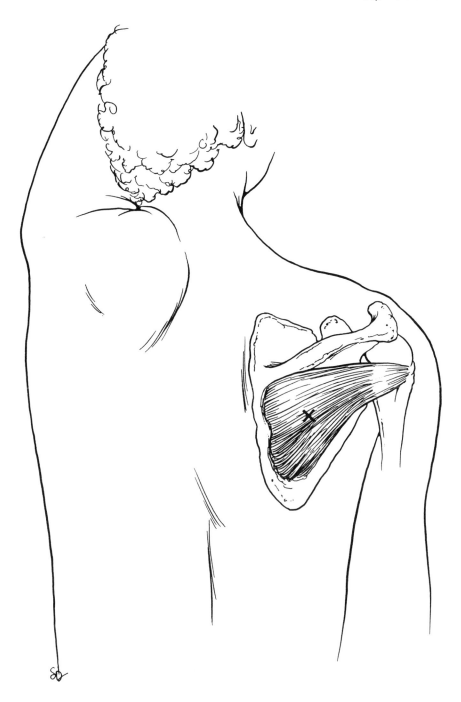

Latissimus Dorsi

PERIPHERAL NERVE   Thoracodorsal (middle subscapular)

ROOT LEVELS   C6, <u>C7</u>, C8

PATIENT POSITION   Side-lying, arm resting across chest.

LOCALIZATION   Posterior axillary fold, directly lateral to the inferior tip of the scapula.

ACTIVATION   Extension/adduction of the humerus.

CAUTION   The electrode inserted too superiorly and posteriorly might be in the teres major or minor.

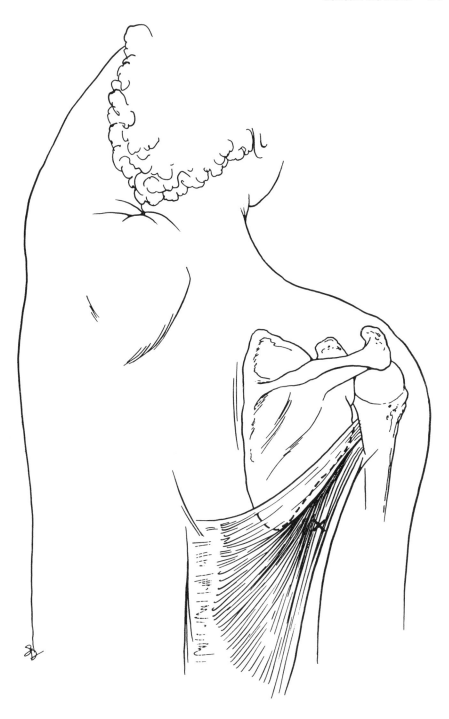

Levator Scapula

PERIPHERAL NERVE   Cervical plexus

ROOT LEVELS   C3, C4, C5

PATIENT POSITION: Prone or side-lying on opposite side.

LOCALIZATION   Midpoint of the line connecting the superior medial scapular border and the nuchal line. Levator scapula is found deep to the overlying upper trapezius.

ACTIVATION   Scapular elevation. Have the patient shrug the shoulder.

CAUTION   Many other muscles, some with similar actions, are in the vicinity of levator scapula, which can therefore be difficult to isolate with certainty. Upper trapezius fibers are found superficially and laterally, splenius capitis and cervicis are deep and medial, and rhomboid minor is at the same depth and inferomedial.

NOTE   Levator scapula frequently receives a contribution from the dorsal scapular nerve, from spinal level C5.

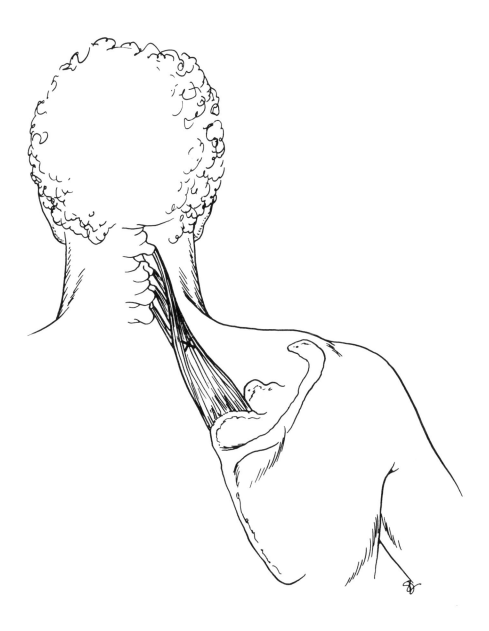

Pectoralis Major

PERIPHERAL NERVE   Medial and lateral pectoral nerves

ROOT LEVELS   C7, C8, T1

PATIENT POSITION   Supine.

LOCALIZATION   Anterior axillary fold, in direct vertical line with the coracoid process.

ACTIVATION   Adduction of the arm.

NOTE   This description is for the sternal portion of the muscle. The clavicular portion is innervated through root levels C5 and C6 primarily; if necessary, it can be reached just inferior to the clavicle, at its midpoint.

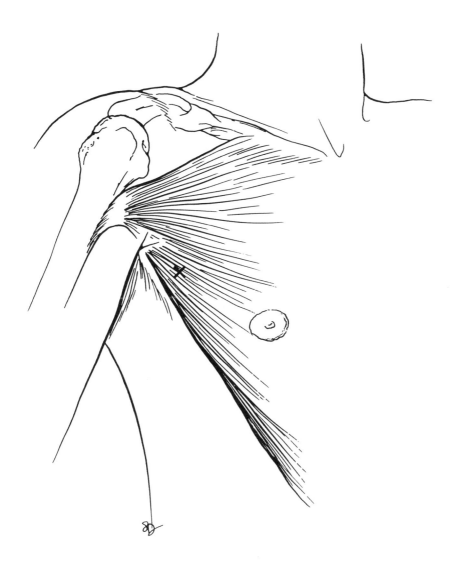

Rhomboid Major

PERIPHERAL NERVE   Dorsal scapular

ROOT LEVELS   C5

PATIENT POSITION   Prone, elbow bent and shoulder internally rotated, so the hand is resting under the abdomen or over the low back.

LOCALIZATION   At the level of the midpoint of the medial scapular border, midway between the border and the high thoracic (T1–T4) spinous processes. The muscle lies deep to middle trapezius.

ACTIVATION   Scapular adduction. Have the patient lift the elbow off the table against resistance.

CAUTION   It can be difficult to differentiate rhomboid major from the more superficial middle trapezius. In well-muscled individuals, the fascial plane between the two muscles can usually be perceived on electrode insertion.

NOTE   The electrode should parallel the muscle fibers, which run at a 45° angle inferolaterally from the upper thoracic spinous processes.

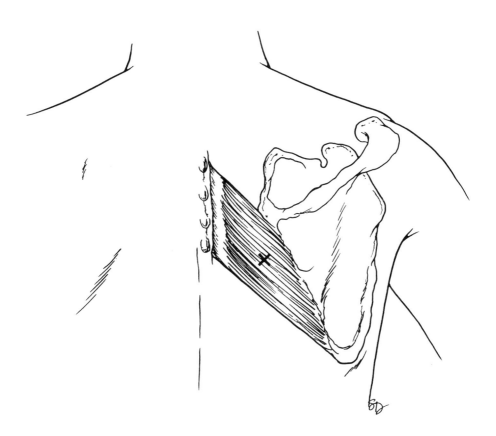

Rhomboid Minor

PERIPHERAL NERVE   Dorsal scapular

ROOT LEVELS   C5

PATIENT POSITION   Prone.

LOCALIZATION   Midpoint of the line connecting the superior medial scapular border and the cervical prominence. Middle trapezius fibers overlie rhomboid minor.

ACTIVATION   Scapular adduction. Have the patient move the scapulae closer together.

CAUTION   Given their proximity and similar functions, rhomboid minor and middle trapezius can be difficult to distinguish electromyographically. In well-muscled individuals, a fascial plane is usually felt as the electrode passes between the two.

NOTE   The electrode should parallel the muscle fibers, which are oriented at an angle of at least 45° from the lower cervical spinous processes inferolaterally to the superior medial scapular border.

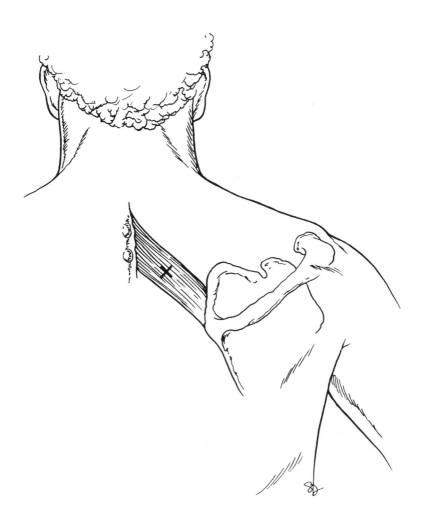

Serratus Anterior

PERIPHERAL NERVE   Long thoracic

ROOT LEVELS   C5, C6, C7

PATIENT POSITION   Lying on opposite side, arm adducted across chest.

LOCALIZATION   In the mid or anterior axillary line, isolate one rib by placing two fingers in the adjacent interspaces, anterior to the bulk of the latissimus dorsi but posterior to the breast tissue in a woman. Needle electrode insertion is directly between your fingers, as serratus anterior is the only muscle between the skin and the rib.

ACTIVATION   Elevation and reaching forward with the arm, i.e., scapular protraction. Providing resistance is sometimes necessary.

CAUTION   Keep your fingers in place during the examination to avoid needle slippage and possible pneumothorax, which has been reported.

NOTE   1. This approach is more reliable than at the muscle origin at the inferior medial scapular border, where it is not easily distinguished from neighboring muscles.
2. The long thoracic nerve is formed directly from the anterior spinal roots. Studying serratus anterior might therefore be helpful in differentiating proximal brachial plexus from root lesions.

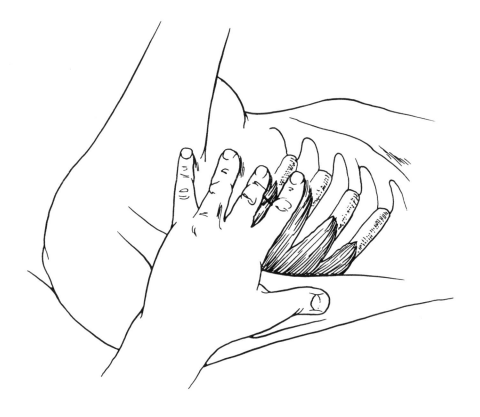

Supraspinatus

PERIPHERAL NERVE	Suprascapular
ROOT LEVELS	<u>C5</u>, C6
PATIENT POSITION	Prone or lying on opposite side, arm relaxed at the side.
LOCALIZATION	At the medial one-third of the scapular spine, insert the electrode immediately superior to the scapular spine. Aim the electrode perpendicular to the skin (not parallel to it) into the depth of the supraspinous fossa, where only supraspinatus is encountered. The aponeurosis of the lateral trapezius fibers is pierced first.
ACTIVATION	Arm abduction.
CAUTION	Pneumothorax has been reported after needle EMG examination of supraspinatus. Be certain to direct the electrode toward the depth of the suprascapular fossa, not in a horizontal plane, so that the apex of the lung is avoided even in cachectic individuals.

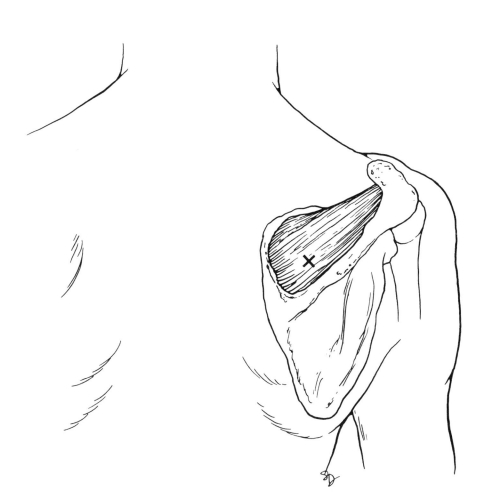

Teres Major

PERIPHERAL NERVE   Lower subscapular

ROOT LEVELS   C5, C6

PATIENT POSITION   Side-lying on opposite side, or prone.

LOCALIZATION   Immediately lateral to the lower one-third of the lateral scapular border.

ACTIVATION   Internal rotation of the arm.

CAUTION   Accompanying teres major at its inferior border is latissimus dorsi, a powerful muscle carrying similar functions.

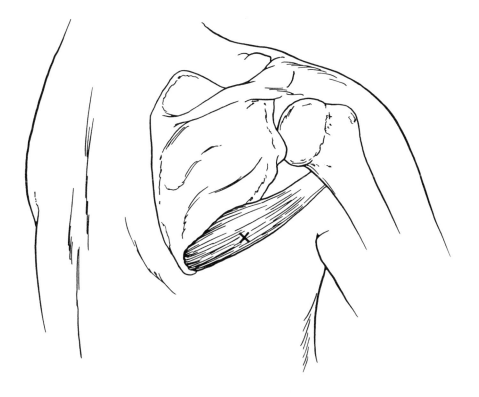

Teres Minor

PERIPHERAL NERVE	Axillary
ROOT LEVELS	<u>C5</u>, C6
PATIENT POSITION	Side-lying on opposite side, or prone.
LOCALIZATION	Immediately lateral to the middle third of the lateral scapular border.
ACTIVATION	External rotation of the arm.
CAUTION	1. Accompanying teres minor at its superior border is infraspinatus, with similar actions but different peripheral nerve supply (suprascapular). 2. In its distal half, beyond the insertion point recommended here, teres minor is covered by fibers of posterior deltoid. That portion of deltoid also causes humeral external rotation.
NOTE	Teres minor denervation can help confirm an axillary mononeuropathy, along with careful study of the three portions of deltoid.

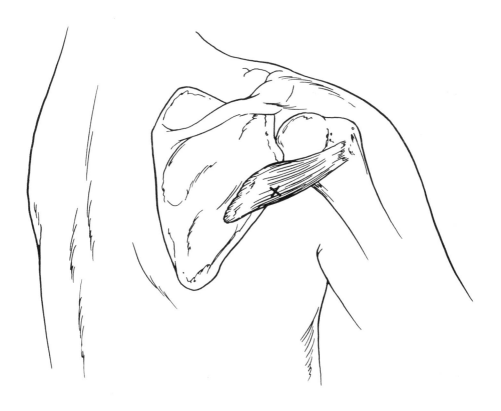

Trapezius, Middle

PERIPHERAL NERVE   Spinal accessory, cervical (subtrapezial) plexus

ROOT LEVELS   Cranial nerve XI, C3, C4

PATIENT POSITION   Prone.

LOCALIZATION   Directly medial to the medial edge of the scapular spine. Keep the electrode superficial, just under the subcutaneous tissue.

ACTIVATION   Scapular adduction.

CAUTION   If the needle is inserted too deeply, it will be in the rhomboid minor, which also causes scapular adduction.

NOTE   On electrode insertion, particularly in well-muscled individuals, one can sometimes feel the fascial plane between the trapezius and rhomboid.

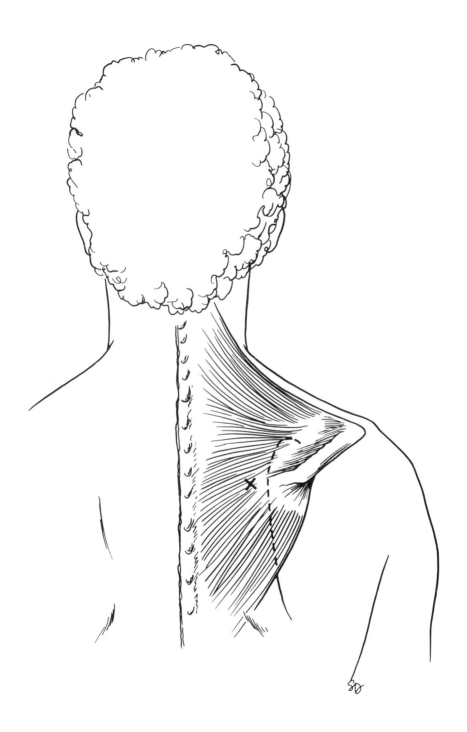

Trapezius, Upper

PERIPHERAL NERVE   Spinal accessory, cervical (subtrapezial) plexus

ROOT LEVELS   Cranial nerve XI, C3, C4

PATIENT POSITION   Side-lying, arm at side.

LOCALIZATION   Superior border of the shoulder, immediately medial to the acromioclavicular joint. The free border of the upper trapezius can be grasped between two fingers at this point, and the electrode parallels the slope of the shoulder.

ACTIVATION   Shoulder elevation. Have the patient shrug the shoulder.

CAUTION   Avoid inserting the needle too far medially, toward the base of the neck. At that point, it could encounter levator scapula.

NOTE   Some controversy exists about whether the innervation from the cervical plexus, C3 and C4, is proprioceptive only or also motor. Most anatomists believe that motor function to the trapezius is purely or primarily supplied by the spinal accessory nerve.

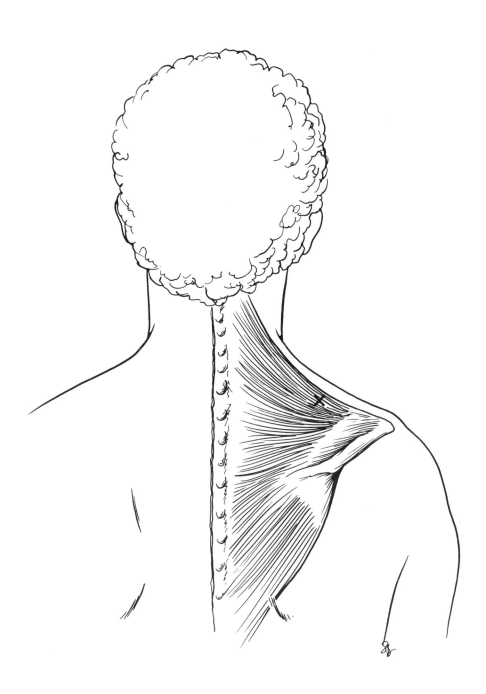

Triceps, Lateral Head

PERIPHERAL NERVE   Radial

ROOT LEVELS   C7, C8

PATIENT POSITION   Supine, forearm across the body, with the elbow resting on the table.

LOCALIZATION   Distal one-third of arm, directly in line with lateral epicondyle, and superficial.

ACTIVATION   Elbow extension.

CAUTION   If the electrode is too anterior, it will be in the most proximal fibers of brachioradialis.

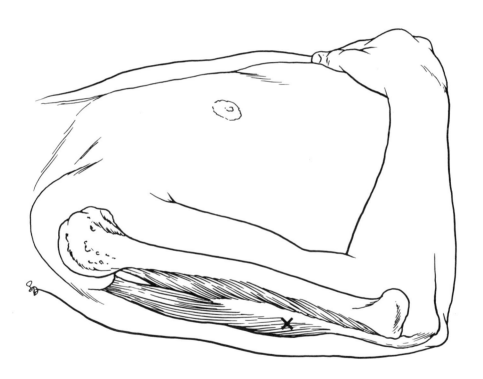

Triceps, Long Head

PERIPHERAL NERVE   Radial

ROOT LEVELS   C7, C8

PATIENT POSITION   Supine, arm adducted across chest.

LOCALIZATION   At the level of the midshaft of the humerus, the electrode is inserted just medial to the posterior midline of the arm.

ACTIVATION   Elbow extension.

CAUTION   1. At this level, the medial head of triceps is deep and medial to the long head, wrapped around the humeral shaft.
2. The lateral head of triceps is located on the lateral one-half of the posterior arm, i.e., across the posterior midline from long head.

NOTE   If the medial head of triceps is to be studied separately, the arm should be abducted away from the body with the shoulder in external rotation. At the level of the humeral midshaft, the needle is inserted at the medial border of the arm, immediately posterior to the neurovascular bundle.

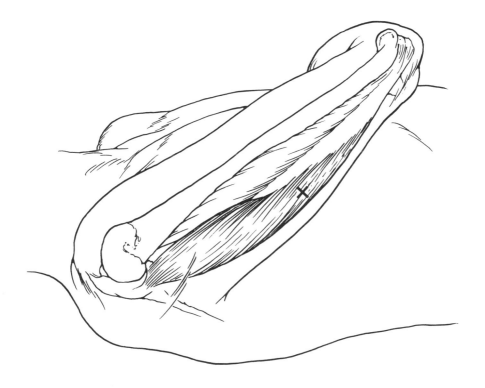

THE
LEG
AND
FOOT

Abductor Digiti Quinti (foot)

PERIPHERAL NERVE	Lateral plantar branch of tibial nerve
ROOT LEVELS	S1, S2
PATIENT POSITION	Supine, leg internally rotated.
LOCALIZATION	At the lateral border of the foot, locate the base of the fifth metatarsal bone, the prominence of which is easily felt. The electrode is inserted immediately proximal to and to the plantar side of the prominence, parallel to the long axis of the foot.
ACTIVATION	Small toe abduction. Ask the patient to fan the toes. Voluntary activation of this muscle can be difficult.
CAUTION	If the needle is inserted too deeply, it could be in the flexor digiti quinti or flexor digitorum brevis, with identical innervations.
NOTE	The abductor digiti quinti is superficial and therefore somewhat susceptible to accumulated trauma. If a foot intrinsic muscle is studied as part of a screen for axonal polyneuropathy, consider the first dorsal interosseous, which lies sheltered between the first two metatarsal bones.

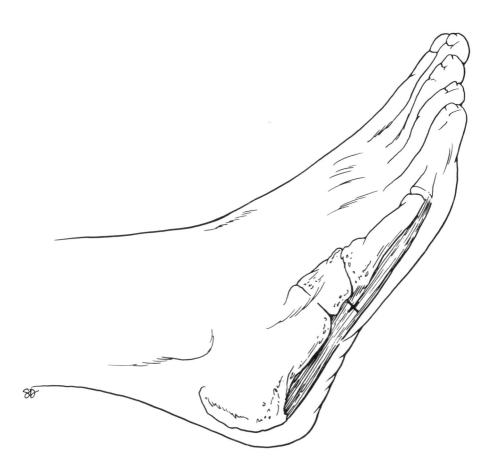

Abductor Hallucis

PERIPHERAL NERVE	Medial plantar branch of tibial nerve
ROOT LEVELS	S1, S2
PATIENT POSITION	Supine, leg externally rotated.
LOCALIZATION	Halfway between the prominence of the navicular bone and the plane of the sole, where it is the most superficial muscle. Insert the electrode parallel to the long axis of the foot.
ACTIVATION	Can be difficult. Ask the patient to fan or curl the toes.
NOTE	Abductor hallucis, being superficial, is susceptible to local trauma. The isolated presence of scattered fibrillation potentials in abductor hallucis should not be taken as significant. The first dorsal interosseous of the foot is a good alternative muscle to screen for polyneuropathy, being both more distal and less susceptible to local trauma than abductor hallucis.

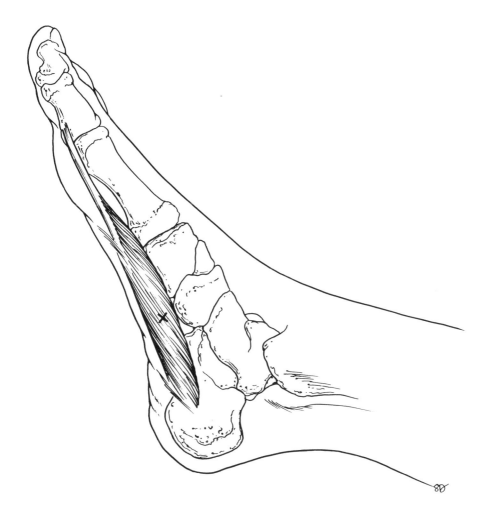

Anterior Tibialis

PERIPHERAL NERVE   Deep branch of peroneal nerve

ROOT LEVELS   L4, L5

PATIENT POSITION   Supine.

LOCALIZATION   At the junction of the middle and upper thirds of the leg, one-quarter of the distance from the tibial shaft to the lateral border of the leg. In this location, it is the only muscle encountered.

ACTIVATION   Ankle dorsiflexion. The patient will sometimes reflexively extend the toes in the same motion, and extensor digitorum longus can substitute for anterior tibialis in producing ankle dorsiflexion. If necessary, hold the toes in plantarflexion while the patient dorsiflexes the ankle.

CAUTION   A needle placed too laterally can be in extensor digitorum longus.

NOTE   There is controversy about the degree of L4 innervation to the anterior tibialis. While some research studies suggest a significant contribution of L4, many clinical electromyographers feel that L5 is the predominant root.

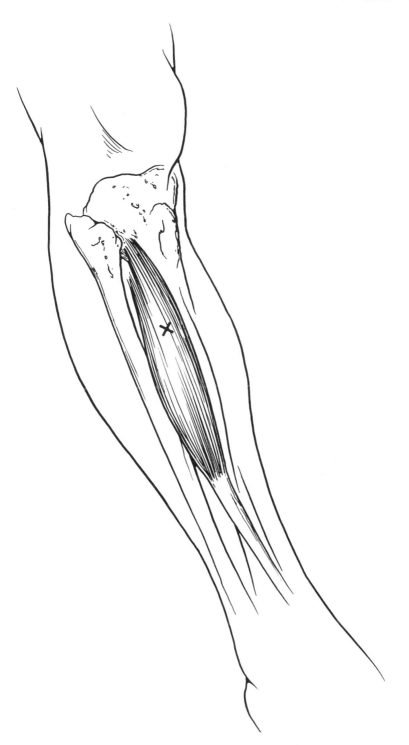

Extensor Digitorum Longus

PERIPHERAL NERVE   Deep branch of peroneal nerve

ROOT LEVELS   L5, S1

PATIENT POSITION   Supine.

LOCALIZATION   At the junction of the upper and middle thirds of the leg, halfway between the tibial shaft and lateral border of the leg. At this point, extensor digitorum longus is the first muscle encountered.

ACTIVATION   Extension of digits 2 through 5.

CAUTION   The needle placed too anteriorly will be in anterior tibialis. If the insertion point is correct but the electrode is directed too deeply, extensor hallucis longus may be entered.

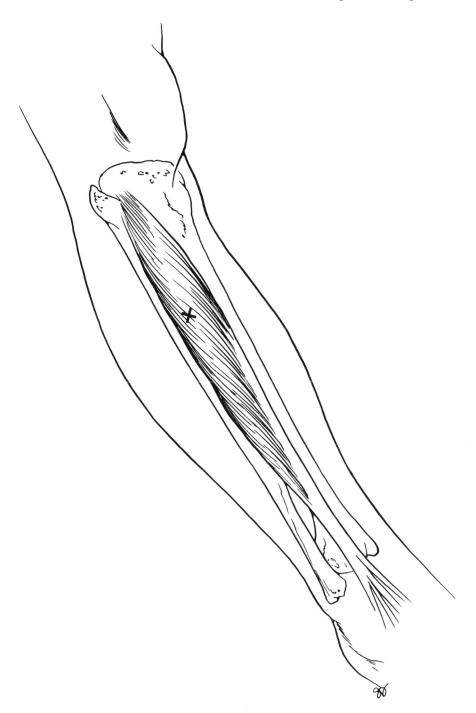

Extensor Hallucis Longus

PERIPHERAL NERVE   Deep branch of peroneal nerve

ROOT LEVELS   L5, S1

PATIENT POSITION   Supine.

LOCALIZATION   At the junction of the middle and lower thirds of the leg, one-third of the distance from the tibial shaft to the lateral border of the leg. The electrode is directed deep and medially.

ACTIVATION   Great toe extension; be certain the needle is pulled back into the subcutaneous tissue before the patient contracts this muscle.

CAUTION   1. The needle inserted or directed too laterally could be in extensor digitorum longus, still partly muscular at this distal location.
2. The deepest fibers of extensor hallucis longus lie against the interosseous membrane, beyond which is posterior tibialis.

NOTE   The belly of extensor hallucis longus is somewhat vertically oriented. The approach recommended here will direct the electrode through the muscle from its side, making it difficult to miss. Additionally, the tendon of anterior tibialis, which is thick at this distal level, will be avoided.

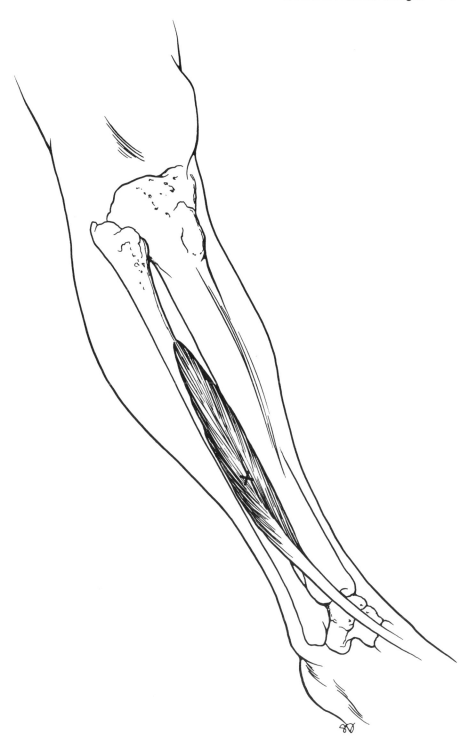

First Dorsal Interosseous (foot)

PERIPHERAL NERVE Lateral plantar branch of tibial nerve

ROOT LEVELS S1, S2

PATIENT POSITION Supine.

LOCALIZATION Place your index finger in the dorsal web space between the first and second toes, pointing distally. Pull your finger proximal until it wedges between the first two metatarsal heads. Insert the electrode immediately distal to your finger and angle it slightly toward the second toe. The muscle is at the depth of the metatarsals; no other muscle is encountered.

ACTIVATION Have the patient curl or fan the toes. Many cannot voluntarily activate the first dorsal interosseous.

CAUTION This muscle is often atrophic in chronic neurogenic conditions. The electrode can then be moved too ventrally and will approach the intrinsic muscles on the flexor side of the foot.

NOTE Needle examination of the foot interosseous muscles is probably the most sensitive indicator of early, distal motor denervation. Buried in the web spaces, these muscles are not as subject to local trauma as abductor hallucis and extensor digitorum brevis.

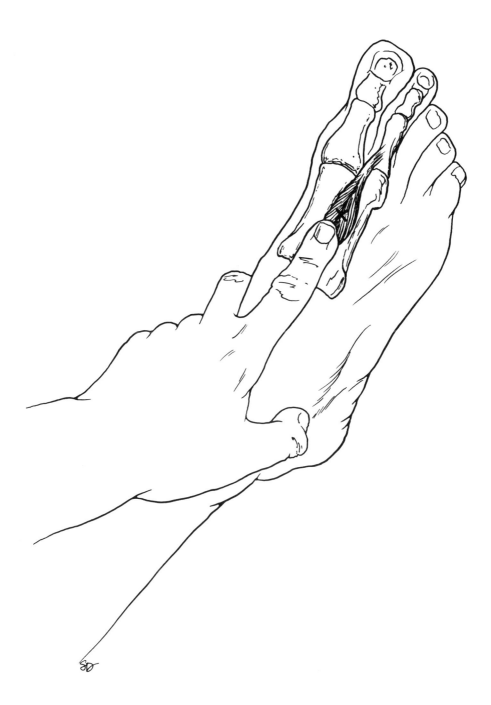

Gastrocnemius, Lateral Head

PERIPHERAL NERVE	Tibial
ROOT LEVELS	S1, S2
PATIENT POSITION	Side-lying on opposite side, or prone.
LOCALIZATION	Midway between the fibular head and the posterior midline of the leg, and superficial.
ACTIVATION	Ankle plantarflexion.
CAUTION	Although lateral gastrocnemius is fairly thick, the electrode inserted too deeply can easily be in the soleus, which is quite a bit thicker.
NOTE	In the supine position, medial gastrocnemius is readily available for needle examination at the medial border of the leg. The medial head is therefore more routinely used than lateral in lower-extremity EMG studies.

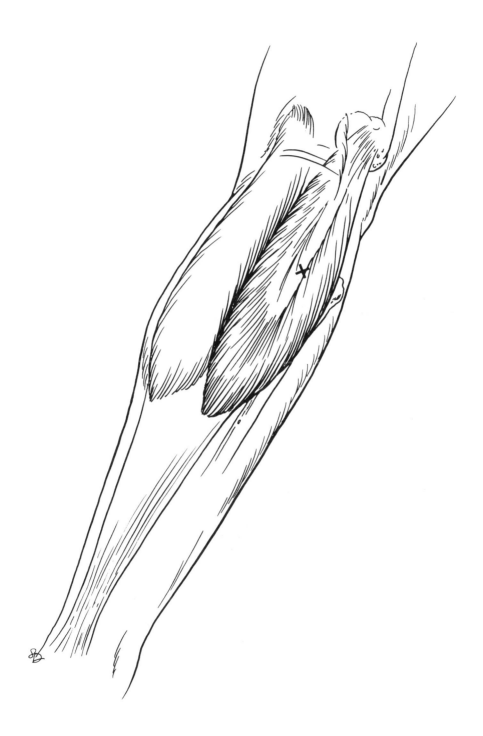

Gastrocnemius, Medial Head

PERIPHERAL NERVE   Tibial

ROOT LEVELS   L5, S1, S2

PATIENT POSITION   Supine.

LOCALIZATION   Medial border of the leg, junction of the upper and middle thirds, and superficial.

ACTIVATION   Ankle plantarflexion.

CAUTION   If the needle is inserted too anteriorly (i.e., closer to the undersurface of the tibia) or too deeply, it could be in soleus.

NOTE   Medial gastrocnemius can be difficult to contract voluntarily because it is quite powerful and because soleus, immediately beneath, carries the same action, is a one-joint muscle, and is therefore at a better mechanical advantage.

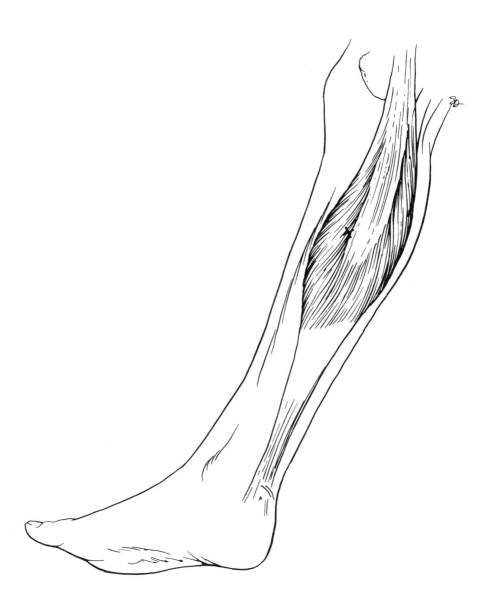

Peroneus Longus

PERIPHERAL NERVE   Superficial branch of peroneal nerve

ROOT LEVELS   L5, S1

PATIENT POSITION   Supine or side-lying.

LOCALIZATION   Straddle the fibular head with your index and middle fingers, pointing proximal. Pull straight down to the junction of the upper and middle thirds of the leg; your fingers will be surrounding peroneus longus, which is the first muscle encountered.

ACTIVATION   Eversion/plantarflexion of the ankle.

CAUTION   The needle directed too anteriorly will enter extensor digitorum longus which, in contrast to peroneus longus, is innervated by the deep branch of the peroneal nerve. Apart from their primary functions, the two muscles can be distinguished as the extensor digitorum longus is an ankle dorsiflexor.

NOTE   The fibular head can be difficult to palpate in the obese patient. In this case, find peroneus longus on the lateral border of the leg, at the junction of the upper and middle thirds.

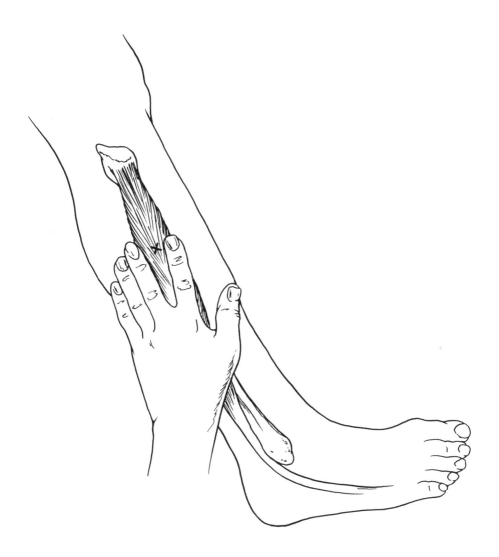

Posterior Tibialis

PERIPHERAL NERVE	Tibial
ROOT LEVELS	L5, S1
PATIENT POSITION	Supine.
LOCALIZATION	There are two acceptable approaches: 1. At the junction of the middle and lower thirds of the leg, insert the electrode under the medial tibial shaft and direct it along the bone and deep, where the muscle lies against the interosseous membrane. The full width of flexor digitorum longus is traversed before posterior tibialis is entered. The illustration depicts this approach. 2. Through anterior tibialis, directly against the lateral border of the tibial shaft, at the junction of the middle and lower thirds of the leg. The electrode crosses the full width of anterior tibialis against the periosteum of the tibia until the interosseous membrane is reached and pierced. Beyond the membrane is posterior tibialis.
ACTIVATION	Plantarflexion/inversion of the ankle.
CAUTION	This is the most deep-lying muscle of the leg and should be avoided on needle examination unless necessary; e.g., posterior tibialis is being considered for tendon transfer.
NOTE	1. Inordinate controversy has arisen about whether posterior tibialis can be reliably reached. The second approach listed is the more reliable if definite placement within this specific muscle is required. With either approach, an electrode longer than the standard 37 mm (1.5 in) will usually be needed. If the standard electrode length is used, the posterior tibialis itself will not be reachable except in very thin individuals. 2. The two approaches start from opposite sides of the tibial shaft, course through an overlying muscle, and then enter essentially the same point of posterior tibialis, i.e., its medial-lying fibers.

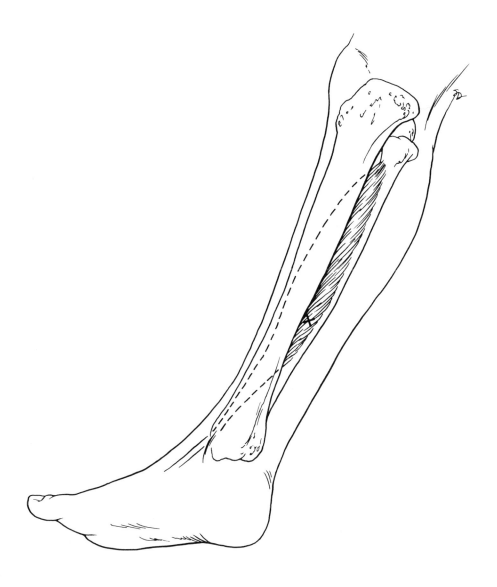

Soleus

PERIPHERAL NERVE   Tibial

ROOT LEVELS   <u>S1</u>, S2

PATIENT POSITION   Prone.

LOCALIZATION   At the junction of the middle and lower thirds of the leg, the needle electrode is inserted immediately adjacent (either medial or lateral) to the posterior midline.

ACTIVATION   Ankle plantarflexion. If the examiner holds the patient's knee in flexion during activation, gastrocnemius contribution to ankle plantarflexion is minimized.

CAUTION   If the needle is placed at the posterior midline or too distal, the tendon of gastrocnemius is encountered first.

NOTE   The muscle bellies of gastrocnemius end abruptly at mid-leg, and in all but obese patients, that landmark can be seen and palpated, facilitating needle localization for soleus. The outline of the muscular portion of gastrocnemius is shown as a dashed line.

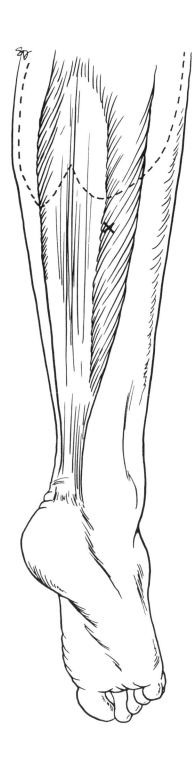

THE
HIP GIRDLE
AND
THIGH

Adductor Longus

PERIPHERAL NERVE   Obturator

ROOT LEVELS   L2, L3, L4

PATIENT POSITION   Supine, thigh slightly abducted and externally rotated.

LOCALIZATION   In the proximal 20% of the thigh, one-quarter the distance from the medial border to the anterior border of the thigh.

ACTIVATION   Thigh adduction.

CAUTION   1. A common mistake is to insert the needle too distally, where adductor longus is no longer superficial.
2. Adductor magnus, partly innervated by the sciatic nerve, can be entered if the electrode is too deep.

NOTE   This muscle is helpful when differentiating an L3 or L4 root lesion or lumbar plexopathy from a femoral mononeuropathy.

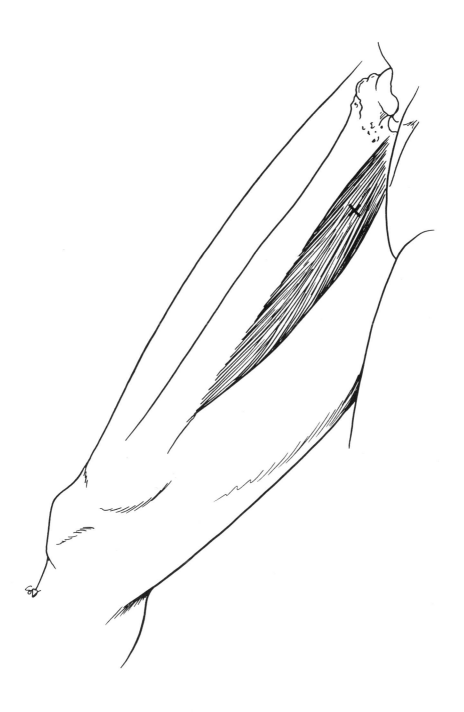

Adductor Magnus

PERIPHERAL NERVE	Obturator and sciatic
ROOT LEVELS	L2, <u>L3</u>, <u>L4</u>
PATIENT POSITION	Supine, thigh externally rotated and abducted.
LOCALIZATION	Upper one-third of thigh, immediately posterior to the medial border of the thigh.
ACTIVATION	Thigh adduction.
CAUTION	If the electrode is inserted or directed too anteriorly, it will be in gracilis. If too posterior, it will be in the medial hamstrings.
NOTE	If muscle definition is good, the posterior edge of gracilis is easily felt. Adductor magnus is then found immediately posterior to gracilis, in the depth of the groove formed by the gracilis edge.

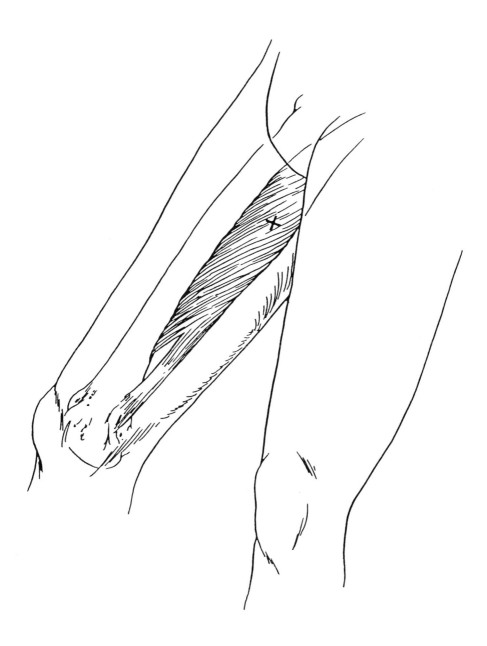

Gluteus Maximus

PERIPHERAL NERVE   Inferior gluteal

ROOT LEVELS   L5, <u>S1</u>, S2

PATIENT POSITION   Prone.

LOCALIZATION   Midpoint of the line connecting the posterior inferior iliac spine and greater trochanter. Gluteus maximus is the first muscle underlying the subcutaneous tissue.

ACTIVATION   Hip extension. Flex the knee to 90° to minimize hip extensor action of the hamstrings, and then have the patient lift the knee off the table. As an alternative, hip abduction.

CAUTION   There are numerous literature reports of injection injury to the sciatic nerve. The nerve, shown in dashed outline, lies medial and distal to the correct insertion point for gluteus maximus.

NOTE   In very obese patients, gluteus maximus can still usually be reached immediately adjacent to and at the superior aspect of the gluteal crease.

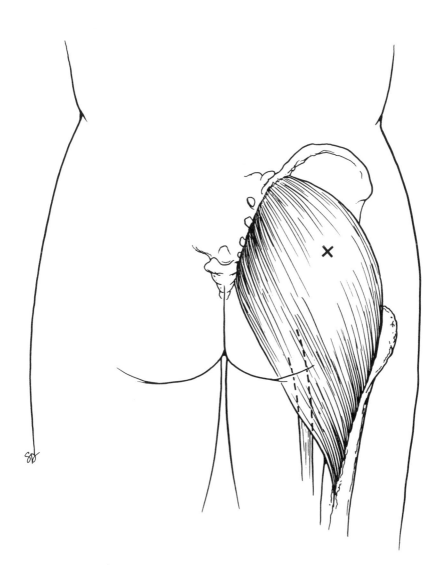

Gluteus Medius

PERIPHERAL NERVE   Superior gluteal

ROOT LEVELS   L4, <u>L5</u>, S1

PATIENT POSITION   Supine.

LOCALIZATION   The anterior border of gluteus medius is defined by the line joining the anterior superior iliac spine (ASIS) and greater trochanter. The electrode is inserted parallel to this line, at its midpoint and just posterior to it. The muscle is the first reached.

ACTIVATION   Internal rotation of the thigh. Needle insertion as described above places it in the anterior fibers of gluteus medius, allowing internal rotation to be used for activation. This motion can be carried out smoothly, as opposed to thigh abduction, which is a cruder motion and which less easily allows for smooth recruitment of motor units.

NOTE   1. The needle placed too anteriorly will be in tensor fascia lata. That muscle, which some practitioners study as a reliable L5 representative, has the same nerve root and peripheral nerve supply as gluteus medius.
2. Gluteus medius is accessible even in the obese patient. The skin is adherent to the ASIS, with little fat overlying, and the muscle can be approached there.

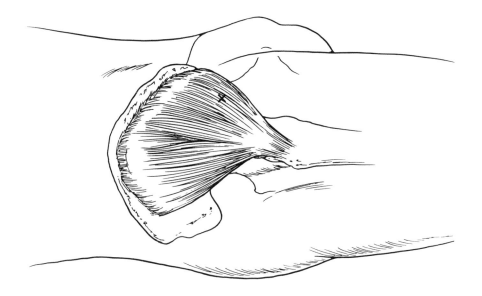

Gracilis

PERIPHERAL NERVE   Obturator

ROOT LEVELS   L2, L3, L4

PATIENT POSITION   Supine, with the thigh externally rotated and abducted.

LOCALIZATION   At the junction of the upper and middle thirds of the thigh, directly medial. At this point, gracilis can usually be surrounded by two fingers, facilitating localization.

ACTIVATION   Thigh adduction.

CAUTION   1. If the needle is too posterior, it will be in adductor magnus, a portion of which is supplied by the sciatic nerve.
2. Needle insertion more distal and too posterior will be in the medial hamstrings, especially semimembranosus.
3. Insertion too distal and anterior will be in a femoral nerve-supplied muscle, either vastus medialis or sartorius.

NOTE   Gracilis and adductor longus are useful in differentiating a lumbar plexopathy or radiculopathy from a pure femoral mononeuropathy.

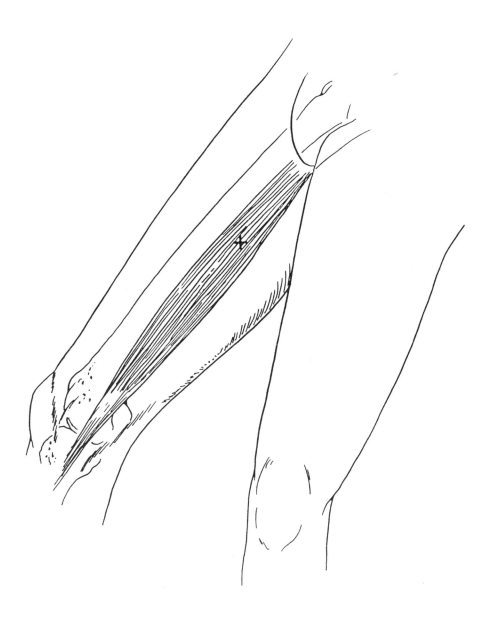

Hamstring External, Biceps Femoris Long Head

PERIPHERAL NERVE   Tibial portion of sciatic nerve

ROOT LEVELS   L5, S1, S2

PATIENT POSITION   Prone.

LOCALIZATION   At midthigh, there is a palpable groove from the iliotibial band between vastus lateralis and the external hamstrings. The needle electrode is inserted just posterior to (i.e., above in the prone position) the groove and parallel to the femur. At this location, the long head is the first muscle reached.

ACTIVATION   Knee flexion; be certain the electrode is first pulled back into subcutaneous tissue. A strongly contracting muscle can easily bend an imbedded EMG electrode.

NOTE   1. The hamstring muscles are more difficult to differentiate when the patient is side-lying, as they tend to droop together toward the table.
2. See the separate description for biceps femoris short head; that muscle is useful in cases of suspected peroneal mononeuropathy at the knee.

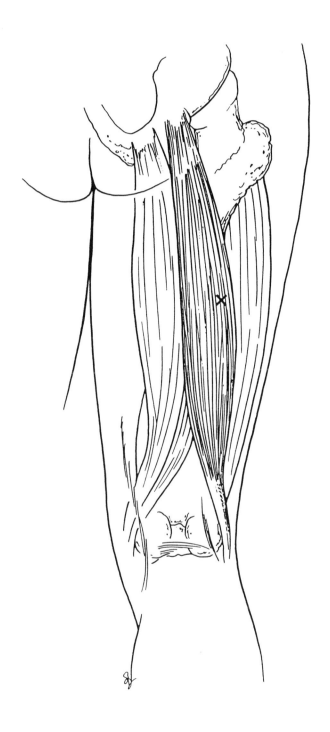

Hamstring External, Biceps Femoris Short Head

PERIPHERAL NERVE   Peroneal portion of sciatic nerve

ROOT LEVELS   L5, <u>S1</u>

PATIENT POSITION   Prone. Place a pillow under the ankles for relaxation if needed.

LOCALIZATION   At the level of the superior crease of the popliteal fossa, immediately medial or lateral to the tendon of biceps femoris long head. The electrode is directed down and under the tendon. At this distal level, long head is tendinous and short head is muscular. The tendon of the long head is shown in dashed outline.

ACTIVATION   Knee flexion.

CAUTION   A common mistake is to insert the needle too proximal, where long head and short head are both muscular. There, the peroneal-innervated short head is not as reliably distinguished from the sciatic-innervated long head.

NOTE   Short head of biceps femoris is usually only examined when localizing a peroneal nerve injury to the region of the fibular head, in which situation short head is spared from denervation.

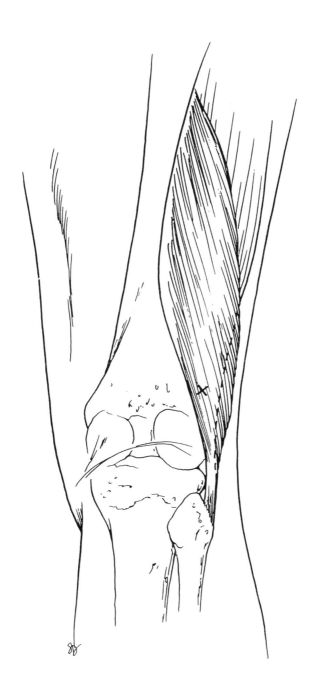

Hamstring Internal, Semimembranosus and Semitendinosus

PERIPHERAL NERVE   Tibial portion of sciatic nerve

ROOT LEVELS   L4, <u>L5</u>, S1, S2

PATIENT POSITION   Prone.

LOCALIZATION   At mid-thigh, at or just medial to the midline and immediately subcutaneous.

ACTIVATION   Knee flexion.

CAUTION   Pull the electrode fully into the subcutaneous tissue before the patient activates this muscle, as the strongly contracting hamstring can bend an electrode embedded in it.

NOTE   If the patient has difficulty relaxing the hamstring muscles during study of insertional activity, place a pillow under the ankles.

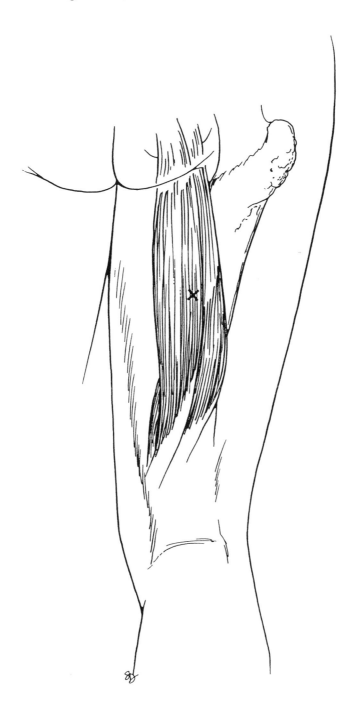

Iliopsoas

PERIPHERAL NERVE	Femoral
ROOT LEVELS	L2, L3
PATIENT POSITION	Supine.
LOCALIZATION	Immediately distal to the inguinal ligament, halfway between the femoral artery pulse and the anterior superior iliac spine. The electrode is directed laterally, away from the neurovascular bundle.
ACTIVATION	Hip flexion.
CAUTION	The femoral artery is illustrated in outline; the femoral nerve is immediately lateral to it. Both lie medial to the point of correct needle insertion.
NOTE	The iliacus portion of the muscle is examined with this approach.

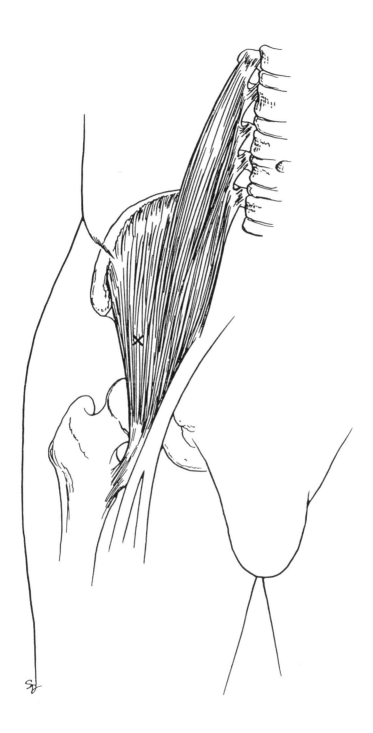

Quadriceps, Rectus Femoris

PERIPHERAL NERVE	Femoral
ROOT LEVELS	L2, L3, L4
PATIENT POSITION	Supine.
LOCALIZATION	At the midpoint of the line connecting the anterior superior iliac spine (ASIS) and the superior pole of the patella. This places the electrode insertion slightly lateral to the geographic center of the anterior thigh.
ACTIVATION	Knee extension.
CAUTION	The muscle becomes thin and eventually tendinous in the distal thigh.
NOTE	1. Except in very obese individuals, rectus femoris is easily outlined by palpation on the anterior thigh.
	2. Sartorius is found along the same line but much more proximally, i.e., immediately distal to the ASIS. Sartorius is also supplied by the femoral nerve.

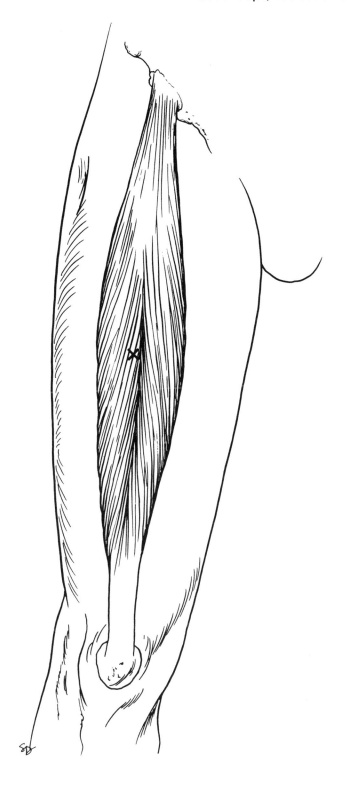

Quadriceps, Vastus Lateralis

PERIPHERAL NERVE   Femoral

ROOT LEVELS   L2, L3, L4

PATIENT POSITION   Supine.

LOCALIZATION   Mid-thigh, directly lateral. In most patients there is a visible and palpable groove between the external hamstring group and vastus lateralis, caused by the iliotibial band. The needle is therefore inserted just anterior to (i.e., above in the supine position) the groove.

ACTIVATION   Knee extension. Have the patient push the back of the knee down into the table or into your hand. Alternatively, have the patient lift the entire leg off the table with the knee straight.

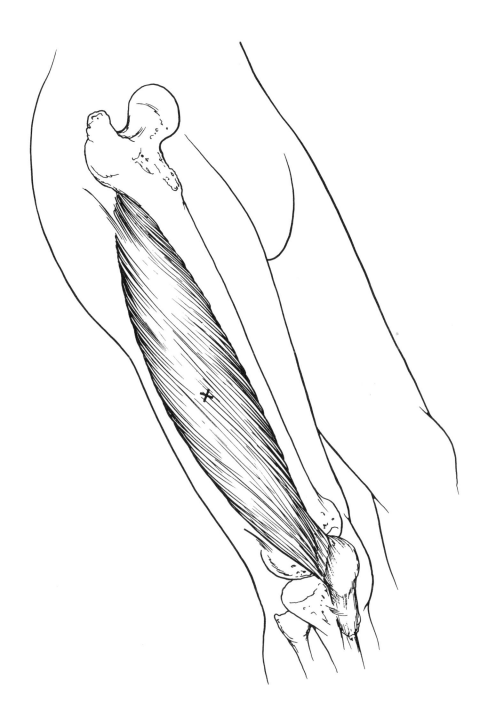

Quadriceps, Vastus Medialis

PERIPHERAL NERVE   Femoral

ROOT LEVELS   L2, L3, L4

PATIENT POSITION   Supine.

LOCALIZATION   The distal 20% of the medial thigh. At this level, the oblique fibers of vastus medialis are angled at nearly 45° toward the patella, and the electrode should parallel them.

ACTIVATION   Knee extension. Have the patient push the back of the knee into the table or your hand. If necessary, have the patient lift the leg off the table with the knee straight and the thigh in external rotation.

CAUTION   If electrode insertion is too proximal and too posterior, it could be in the medial hamstring or adductor magnus, innervated by different nerves.

NOTE   In the very thin or cachectic patient, vastus medialis is often underdeveloped or atrophic. Choose vastus lateralis in that situation.

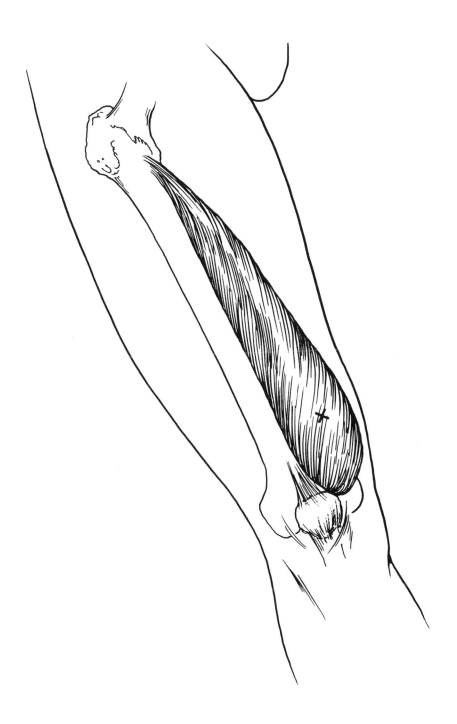

THE
NON-LIMB
MUSCLES

Anal Sphincter

PERIPHERAL NERVE	Inferior rectal branch of pudendal nerve
ROOT LEVELS	S2, S3, <u>S4</u>
PATIENT POSITION	Side-lying, with the uppermost hip in full flexion.
LOCALIZATION	With a gloved finger in the rectum, insert the electrode at the mucocutaneous junction, and angle it toward your finger.
ACTIVATION	Ask the patient to tighten the sphincter around your finger. Relaxation is best obtained by having the patient strain, simulating pushing to have a bowel movement.
CAUTION	Always advance the electrode slowly and use the gloved finger to "feel" the approaching needle electrode, thereby avoiding piercing the rectal wall.
NOTE	1. The anal sphincter can be studied bilaterally, or in quadrants, to gain information about sacral or central cauda equina lesions. 2. With the index finger in the rectum, the thumb and middle digit of the same hand are usually needed to separate the gluteal tissue, to allow visualization for proper needle insertion.

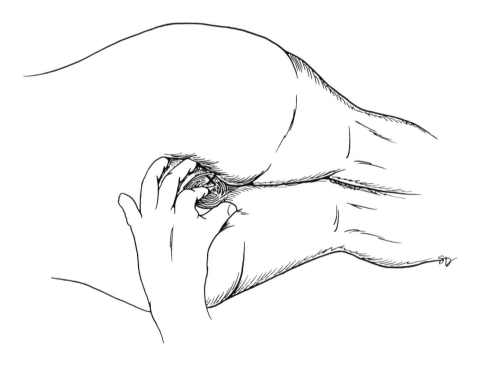

Diaphragm

PERIPHERAL NERVE	Phrenic
ROOT LEVELS	C3, <u>C4</u>, C5
PATIENT POSITION	Supine.
LOCALIZATION	Anterior axillary line, eighth or ninth rib interspace. The intercostal muscles are encountered first, then the diaphragm, identified by its cyclic contractions with breathing. If there are no voluntary contractions originating from the diaphragm, correct localization relies on recognizing that the first insertional activity heard is from the intercostal muscles, followed by an electrically silent gap, then the insertional activity from the targeted muscle.
ACTIVATION	Respiration.
CAUTION	At this level, the pleural space is avoided. If the electrode is inserted in a more proximal interspace, it is possible to enter the pleural space, with some risk of causing pneumothorax.
NOTE	If for some reason this approach is not feasible, approach the diaphragm from the costal margin at the midclavicular line. With the patient supine, depress the abdominal contents with one hand and direct the electrode superiorly and along the underside of the ribs. The origin of the abdominal muscles will be encountered first, then a gap, then the diaphragm. This approach tends to be uncomfortable and is technically impossible in the obese patient.

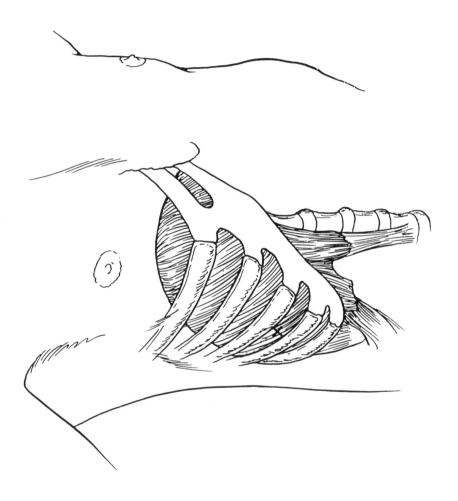

Orbicularis Oculi

PERIPHERAL NERVE   Temporal and zygomatic branches of facial nerve

ROOT LEVELS   Cranial nerve VII

PATIENT POSITION   Supine.

LOCALIZATION   Two-thirds the distance from the anterior border of the ear to the lateral edge of the orbit. From that point, direct the electrode toward the lateral canthus of the eye and remain superficial.

ACTIVATION   Closing or squeezing of the eyelids.

CAUTION   The muscles of facial expression are extremely thin, and the electrode must remain quite superficial.

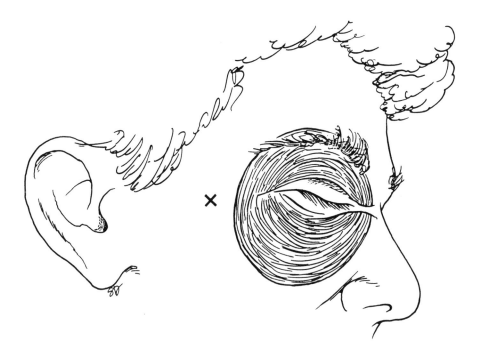

Orbicularis Oris

PERIPHERAL NERVE   Buccal branches of facial nerve

ROOT LEVELS   Cranial nerve VII

PATIENT POSITION   Supine.

LOCALIZATION   Two-thirds the distance from the angle of the jaw to the corner of the mouth. From that point, direct the electrode toward the corner of the mouth and remain superficial.

ACTIVATION   Whistling motion of the lips.

CAUTION   The muscles of facial expression are extremely thin, and the electrode must remain quite superficial.

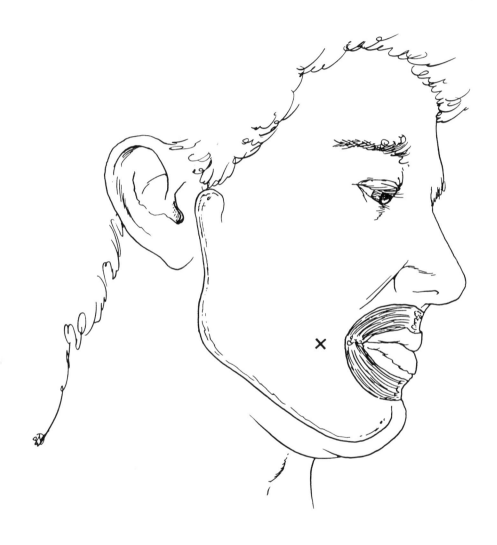

Paraspinals, Cervical (Erector Spinae)

PERIPHERAL NERVE   Posterior primary rami

ROOT LEVELS   C1 through T1

PATIENT POSITION   Prone, with the neck flexed over a pillow placed under the upper chest, and the arms by the sides. Alternatively, side-lying on the opposite side, neck fully flexed and supported by a pillow. The shoulder should be relaxed with the trapezius quiet and the arm by the side.

LOCALIZATION   Adjacent to the cervical spine, in vertical line with the midpoint of the nuchal ridge. The electrode is inserted perpendicular to the skin and must travel through trapezius before reaching the paraspinals. This transition is usually easily felt and heard, as there is a fascial plane separating the two. The insertion point shown is for the midcervical paraspinal muscles.

ACTIVATION   Gentle isometric neck extension, with the electrode in subcutaneous tissue first.

CAUTION   Pneumothorax has occurred following needle examination of cervical paraspinal muscles in very thin individuals.

NOTE   1. This is perhaps the most difficult group of muscles to relax. Gentle resistance of neck flexion with the examiner's hand is occasionally helpful in relaxing the antagonist, i.e., the paraspinals.
2. There are several other components to the paraspinal group apart from the erector spinae. The splenius capitis and cervicis lie superficial, with the rotatores, multifidus, and interspinales deep against the vertebrae. During electromyography, the electrode is most likely to be in the erector muscles, although the deep group carries less root level overlap.

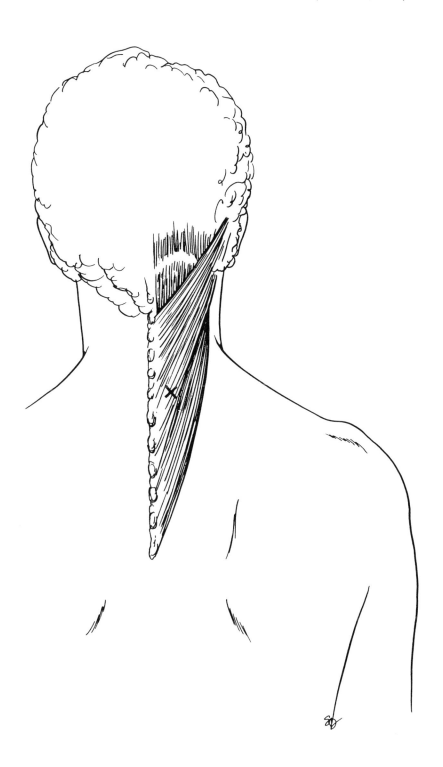

Paraspinals, Lumbosacral (Erector Spinae)

PERIPHERAL NERVE	Posterior primary rami
ROOT LEVELS	L1 through S1, (S2)
PATIENT POSITION	Prone.
LOCALIZATION	The point halfway between the posterior superior iliac spine and the midline corresponds to the low lumbar paraspinal muscles. Needle electrode insertion for more proximal or distal levels is through the same point and along the line parallel to the spine. The electrode is directed perpendicular to the skin and somewhat medially, toward the deeper paraspinal layers.
ACTIVATION	Hip extension. This will secondarily cause the paraspinal muscles to contract.
CAUTION	Make certain the needle is in subcutaneous tissue before asking for a voluntary contraction. Study voluntary motor units only if this is important in the overall electrodiagnostic picture; it often is not.
NOTE	1. Lumbosacral paraspinal muscles are easily relaxed if the patient is prone, and both sides can be examined without changing position. In the side-lying position, these muscles are more difficult to relax, particularly on the side closer to the table. 2. To facilitate relaxation of these muscles to study insertional activity, have the patient push the small of the back up against your fingers. This is the same motion performed in a pelvic tilt exercise. 3. S1 is definitely represented in the paraspinals. Controversy exists about S2; if there is S2 representation, it is likely inconsistent and incomplete. 4. When possible, examine the deeper layers of the paraspinal muscles, because less root level overlap occurs there.

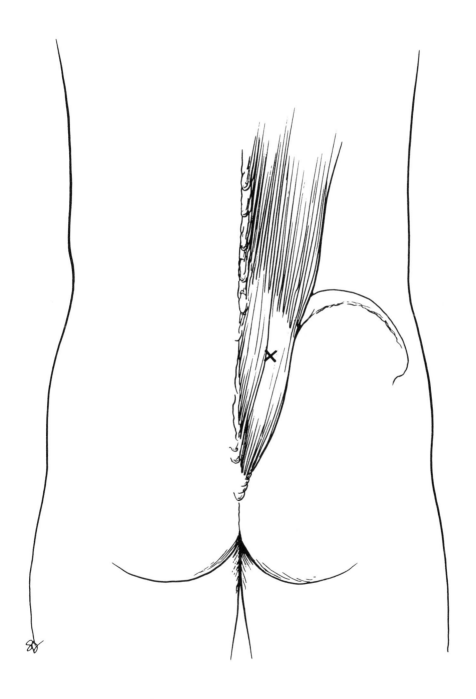

Sternocleidomastoid

PERIPHERAL NERVE	Spinal accessory, cervical plexus
ROOT LEVELS	Cranial nerve XI, C2, C3
PATIENT POSITION	Supine, with the head turned to the contralateral side.
LOCALIZATION	Midway between the mastoid and clavicular attachments of the muscle. Enter it from its lateral side and parallel to its course.
ACTIVATION	Have the patient turn the head to the opposite side, against your hand.
NOTE	The spinal accessory nerve is sometimes damaged during lymph node dissection in the posterior triangle of the neck, affecting trapezius. The sternocleidomastoid will be spared from denervation in this situation, and its examination may prove helpful for localization of the lesion.

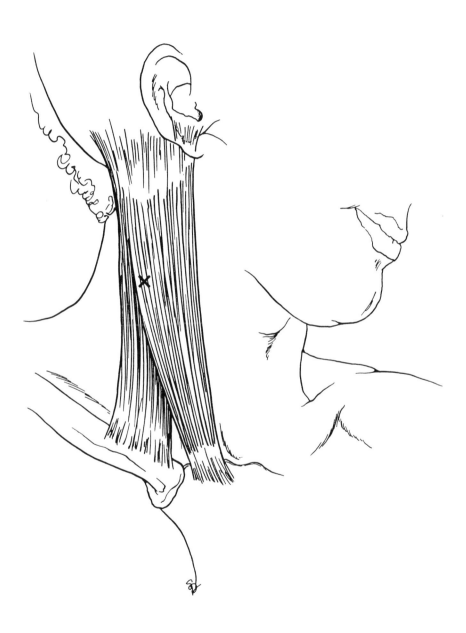

Tongue (Genioglossus)

PERIPHERAL NERVE   Hypoglossal

ROOT LEVELS   Cranial nerve XII

PATIENT POSITION   Supine, head tilted slightly into extension.

LOCALIZATION   Midpoint between tip of chin and the angle of the jaw, medial to the mandible. The tongue is found deep here, after the electrode passes through mylohyoid and geniohyoid muscles.

ACTIVATION   Protraction of the tongue. Ask the patient to stick out the tongue.

NOTE   1. Alternatively, the patient's tongue can be grasped with a gauze pad and the inferolateral portion examined. Relaxation in order to study insertional activity requires retraction of the tongue, which is difficult with the needle in place.
2. Genioglossus is one of five extrinsic tongue muscles controlling movement; the others are hyo-, chondro-, stylo-, and palato-glossus. Genioglossus lies most inferior and is therefore most likely to be reached with the electrode.

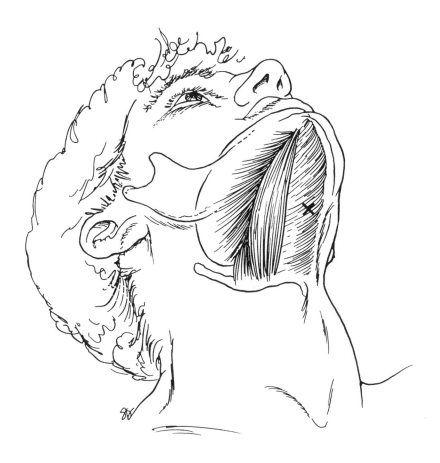

Index